Obstetric Clinical Algorithms: Management and Evider

Obstetric Clinical Algorithms: Management and Evidence

Errol R. Norwitz MD PhD

Professor, Yale University School of Medicine
Co-Director, Division of Maternal-Fetal Medicine
Director, Maternal-Fetal Medicine Fellowship Program
Director, Obstetrics & Gynecology Residency Program
Department of Obstetrics, Gynecology & Reproductive Sciences
Yale-New Haven Hospital
New Haven, CT, USA

Michael A. Belfort MD PhD

Professor, Department of Obstetrics and Gynecology
University of Utah School of Medicine
Salt Lake City, UT and
Director, Perinatal Research and Fetal Therapy Program
HCA Healthcare, Nashville, TN, USA

George R. Saade MD

Professor, Department of Obstetrics and Gynecology
University of Texas Medical Branch
Galveston, TX, USA

Hugh Miller MD

Department of Obstetrics and Gynecology
University of Arizona
Tucson, AZ, USA

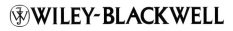

A John Wiley & Sons, Ltd., Publication

This edition first published 2010. © 2010 by E.R. Norwitz, M. Belfort,
G.R. Saade and H. Miller

Blackwell Publishing was acquired by John Wiley & Sons in February 2007. Blackwell's
publishing program has been merged with Wiley's global Scientific, Technical and Medical
business to form Wiley-Blackwell.

Registered office: John Wiley & Sons Ltd, The Atrium, Southern Gate, Chichester, West
Sussex, PO19 8SQ, UK

Editorial offices: 9600 Garsington Road, Oxford, OX4 2DQ, UK
          111 River Street, Hoboken, NJ 07030-5774, USA
          The Atrium, Southern Gate, Chichester, West Sussex, PO19 8SQ, UK

For details of our global editorial offices, for customer services and for information about
how to apply for permission to reuse the copyright material in this book please see our
website at www.wiley.com/wiley-blackwell

The right of the author to be identified as the author of this work has been asserted in
accordance with the Copyright, Designs and Patents Act 1988.

ISBN: 9781405181112

A catalogue record for this book is available from the British Library.

Set in 8.75/12pt Minion by MPS Limited, A Macmillan Company

Printed in Singapore by Markono Print Media Pte Ltd

2   2012

Contents

Preface

Advances in obstetric practice and research over the past several decades have resulted in significant improvements in maternal and perinatal outcome. Such improvements carry with them added responsibility for the obstetric care provider in practice today. The decision to embark on a particular course of management simply because *"that's the way we did it when I was in training"* or because *"it worked the last time I tried it"* is no longer reasonable or justifiable. Clinical decisions should, as far as possible, be evidence based. Evidence-based medicine is defined as *"the conscientious, explicit, and judicious use of current best evidence in making decisions about the care of individual patients"* [1]. This statement requires that obstetric care providers be familiar with all the latest publications, be able to judge the quality of the data being presented (for example, randomized double-blind placebo-controlled clinical trials hold more validity than case reports or expert opinion), and be able to balance the risks and potential benefits of various treatment options.

In practice, evidence-based medicine requires expertise in retrieving, interpreting, and applying the results of scientific studies and in communicating effectively the risks and benefits of different courses of action to patients. This daunting task is compounded by the fact that the volume of medical literature is expanding at more than 7% per annum and doubling every 10-15 years. Even within the relatively narrow field of Obstetrics & Gynecology, there are more than five major publications each month containing an excess of 100 original articles and 35 editorials. How then does a busy practitioner maintain a solid foundation of up-to-date knowledge within the scope of his or her practice and synthesize these data into individual management plans? New information can be gleaned from a variety of sources: the advice of colleagues and consultants, textbooks, lectures and continuing medical education courses, peer-reviewed medical journals with original research articles and reviews, and from published clinical guidelines and consensus statements. The internet has created an additional virtual dimension by allowing instant access to the medical literature to both providers and patients, thereby removing the reliance on clinical experience and expert opinion. It is with this background in mind that we have written *Obstetric Clinical Algorithms: Management and Evidence.*

There is mounting evidence that standardization of management across a wide range of clinical care providers results in a significant reduction in medical errors and improvements in both patient safety and obstetric outcomes [2,3]. The development of standardized obstetric algorithms is one way to achieve this goal. A medical algorithm can best be described as a *finite, logical, step-by-step sequence of instructions or operations for solving a particular clinical problem.* In this text, we use flow diagrams based on best practice to mimic the decision-making processes that go on in our brains when faced with a vexing clinical problem. To further facilitate decision-making, we have superimposed 'levels of evidence' onto the algorithms as defined by the report of the *US Preventive Services Task Force (USPSTF)* of the Agency for Healthcare Research Quality, an independent panel of experts in primary care and prevention appointed and funded by the government of the United States that systematically reviews the evidence of effectiveness and develops recommendations for clinical preventive services [4]. The table below summarizes the 'levels of evidence' used in this text.

'Levels of Evidence' used in *Obstetric Clinical Algorithms: Management and Evidence:*

Color key	Levels of evidence available on which to base recommendations *	Recommendation/ suggestions for practice
Red bold	Level I / II-1	**Definitely offer or provide this service**
Red regular	Level II-1 / II-2	Consider offering or providing this service
Red italics	*Level II-2 / II-3 / III*	*Discuss this service, but insufficient evidence to strongly recommend it*
Black regular	Level II-3 / III	Insufficient evidence to recommend this service, but may be a reasonable option

*Levels of evidence are based on the 'hierarchy of research design' used in the report of the 2nd US Preventive Services Task Force:

Level I: Evidence obtained from at least one properly powered and conducted randomized controlled trial (RCT); also includes well-conducted systematic review or meta-analysis of homogeneous RCTs.

Level II-1: Evidence obtained from well-designed controlled trials without randomization.

Level II-2: Evidence obtained from well-designed cohort or case-control analytic studies, preferably from more than one center or research group.

Level II-3: Evidence obtained from multiple time series with or without the intervention; dramatic results from uncontrolled trials might also be regarded as this type of evidence.

Level III: Opinions of respected authorities, based on clinical experience; descriptive studies or case reports; or reports of expert committees.

Obstetric care providers can be broadly divided into two philosophical or stylistic camps: those who believe that everything possible should be offered in a given clinical setting in the hope that something will help (also called the "*we don't have all the information we need*" group or the "*might as well give it, it won't do any harm*" group) and those who hold out against popular opinion until there is consistent and compelling scientific evidence that an individual course of action is beneficial and has a favorable risk-to-benefit ratio (sometimes referred to as "*therapeutic nihilists*"). As protagonists of the latter camp, we argue that substantial harm can in fact be done—both to individual patients and to society as a whole—by implementing management plans that have not been the subject of rigorous scientific investigation followed by thoughtful introduction into clinical practice. In *Obstetric Clinical Algorithms: Management and Evidence,* we have attempted to provide evidence-based management recommendations for common obstetric conditions. However, individual clinical decisions should not be based on medical algorithms alone, but should be compared with and tempered by clinical knowledge and physician judgment. It is the sincere hope of the authors that the reader will find this book both practical and informative. At all times, the primary focus should be the delivery of a healthy mother and a healthy baby.

Errol R. Norwitz
Michael A. Belfort
George Saade
Hugh Miller

1. Sackett DL, Rosenberg WM, Gray JA et al.. Evidence based medicine: what it is and what it isn't. BMJ 1996;312:71-72.
2. Pettker CM, Thung SF, Norwitz ER et al. Impact of a comprehensive patient safety strategy on obstetric adverse events. Am J Obstet Gynecol 2009;200:492 (e1-8).
3. Clark SL, Belfort MA, Byrum SL et al.. Improved outcomes, fewer cesarean deliveries, and reduced litigation: results of a new paradigm in patient safety. Am J Obstet Gynecol 2008;199:105 (e1-7).
4. Report of the US Preventive Services Task Force (USPSTF). Available at http://www.ahrq.gov/clinic/uspstfix.htm (last accessed on 24 August 2009).

List of abbreviations

✔	Check or confirm	CCAM	congenital cystic adenoid malformation
3TC	lamivudine	CD4	cluster of differentiation 4
ABG	arterial blood gas	CDC	Centers for Disease Control and Prevention in the United States
ACA	anticardiolipin antibody		
ACE	angiotensin-converting enzyme	CF	cystic fibrosis
ACOG	American College of Obstetricians and Gynecologists	CFU	colony-forming units
		CI	cervical insufficiency (previously known as cervical incompetence)
ADH	antidiuretic hormone		
AFE	amniotic fluid embolism	CIN 1	Cervical intraepithelial neoplasia 1
AFI	amniotic fluid index	CL	cervical length
AGA	appropriate for gestational age	CMV	cytomegalovirus
AGUS	abnormal glandular cells of undetermined significance	CNS	central nervous system
		CPD	cephalopelvic disproportion
ALT	alanine transaminase	CPR	cardiopulmonary resuscitation
AMA	advanced maternal age	CSF	cerebrospinal fluid
ANA	antinuclear antibodies	CST	contraction stress test (also known as the oxytocin challenge test (OCT))
APLAS	antiphospholipid antibody syndrome		
ARDS	acute respiratory distress syndrome	CT scan	computerised tomography scan
		CTG	cardiotocography
ART	assisted reproductive technology	CVS	chorionic villus sampling
ASCUS	atypical squamous cells of undetermined significance	CXR	chest x-ray
		D&C	dilatation and curettage
ATP	alloimmune thrombocytopenia	D&E	dilatation and evacuation
AZT	azidothymidine (zidovudine)	D4T	stavudine
BCG vaccination	Bacille Calmette–Guérin vaccination	DDI	didanosine
		DES	diethylstilbestrol
bid	two times a day	Di/di twins	dichorionic-diamniotic twins
BMI	body mass index	DIC	disseminated intravascular coagulopathy
BP	blood pressure		
bpm	beats per minute	DKA	diabetic ketoacidosis
BPP	biophysical profile	DNA	deoxyribonucleic acid
BUN	blood urea nitrogen	dsDNA	double-stranded DNA
BV	bacterial vaginosis	DSM	Diagnostic and Statistical Manual of Mental Disorders
CAGE questionnaire	screening test for problem drinking		
		DVT	deep vein thrombosis
CBC	complete blood count	E. coli	Escherichia coli

EBL	estimated blood loss		**HUS**	hemolytic uremic syndrome
ECC	endocervical curettage		**ICU**	intensive care unit
ECT	electroconvulsant therapy		**ID consult**	infectious disease consult
ECV	external cephalic version		**IgG**	immunoglobulin G
EDD	estimated date of delivery (or the estimated dute date)		**IgM**	immunoglobulin M
			IMI	intramuscular injection
EEG	electroencephalogram		**INH**	isoniazid
EFM	electronic fetal heart rate monitoring		**INR**	International Normalized Ratio
EFW	estimated fetal weight		**IOL**	induction of labor
EKG	electrocardiogram		**IQ**	intelligence quotient
ELISA	enzyme-linked immunosorbant assay		**ITP**	immune thrombocytopenic purpura
EMB	endometrial biopsy			
FDA	Food and Drug Administration of the United States		**IUFD**	intrauterine fetal demise
			IUGR	intrauterine growth restriction
FeNa	fractional excretion of sodium		**IUPC**	intrauterine pressure catheter
FEV1	forced expiratory volume in one second		**IUT**	intrauterine transfusion
			IV	intravenous
fFN	fetal fibronectin		**IVF**	*in vitro* fertilization
FFP	fresh frozen plasma		**IVIG**	intravenous immune globulin
FLM	fetal lung maturity		**K$^+$**	potassium
FSE	fetal scalp electrode		**L&D**	labor & delivery
FTA-ABS	fluorescent treponemal antibody absorption		**LAC**	lupus anticoagulant
			LAIV	live-attenuated viral influenza vaccine
FVC	forced vital capacity			
GBS	group B β-hemolytic streptococcus		**LEEP**	loop electrosurgical excision procedure
GCT	glucose challenge test (also known as glucose load test (GLT))			
			LENI testing	lower extremity noninvasive testing
GDM	gestational diabetes		**LGA**	large-for-gestational age
GFR	glomerular filtration rate		**LGSIL**	low-grade squamous intraepithelial lesions
GLT	glucose load test (also known as a glucose challenge test (GCT))			
			LMP	last menstrual period
GTT	glucose tolerance test		**LMWH**	low molecular weight heparin
HAART	highly-active antiretroviral therapy		**LTL**	laparoscopic tubal ligation
			M. tuberculosis	Mycobacterium tuberculosis
HbA$_{1c}$	haemoglobin A1C		**MCA**	middle cerebral artery
HBIg	hepatitis B immunoglobulin		**MDI**	metered dose inhaler
HBV	hepatitis B virus		**MFM**	maternal-fetal medicine
hCG	human chorionic gonadotropin		**MFPR**	multifetal pregnancy reduction
HCO$_3$	bicarbonate		**MHA-TP**	microhemagglutination assay for antibodies to *T. pallidum*
HEG	hyperemesis gravidarum			
HELLP syndrome	Hemolysis, Elevated Liver enzymes and Low Platelets		**MMR vaccine**	measles, mumps and rubella vaccine
HGSIL	high-grade squamous intraepithelial lesions		**MoM**	multiples of the median
			MRI	magnetic resonance imaging
HIE	hypoxic ischemic encephalopathy		**MS-AFP**	maternal serum α-fetoprotein
HIV	human immunodeficiency virus		**MTX**	Methotrexate
HPV	human papilloma viruses		**Na$^+$**	sodium
HSV	herpes simplex virus		**NDDG**	National Diabetes Data Group

NICHD	National Institute of Child Health and Human Development	**Rh status**	Rhesus antigen status
NICU	neonatal intensive care unit	**RLQ**	right lower quadrant
NIDDM	noninsulin-dependent diabetes mellitus	**R-NST**	reactive NST
		RPR	rapid plasma reagin
NR-NST	nonreactive NST	**RUQ**	right upper quadrant
NS	normal saline	**SC**	subcuticular
NSAID	nonsteroidal anti-inflammatory drugs	**SGA**	small-for-gestational age
		SIADH	syndrome of inappropriate ADH secretion
NST	nonstress testing	**SIDS**	sudden infant death syndrome
NT	nuchal translucency	**SLE**	systemic lupus erythematosus
NTD	neural tube defect	**SSKI**	saturated solution of potassium iodide
NVD	normal vaginal delivery		
NVP	nausea and vomiting in pregnancy	**STI**	sexually transmitted infection
OCT	oxytocin challenge test (also known as the contraction stress test (CST))	**T&S**	type and screen
		T. pallidum	Treponema pallidum
		T_3	triiodithyronine
OR	operating room	T_4	levothyroxine
PAP smear	Papanicolaou test	**TB**	tuberculosis
PAPP-A	pregnancy-associated plasma protein A	**TBG**	thyroxine-binding globulin
		TFT	thyroid function tests
PCO_2	partial pressure of carbon dioxide	**tid**	three times a day
PCOS	polycystic ovary syndrome	**TIV**	trivalent inactivated influenza vaccine
PCP	Pneumocystis carinii pneumonia		
PCR	polymerase chain reaction	**TORCH infections**	toxoplasmosis, rubella, CMV and herpes simplex infections
PE	pulmonary embolism		
PEFR	peak expiratory flow rate	**TPPA**	*T. pallidum* particle agglutination assay
PET	pre-eclamptic toxemia		
PGE_1	prostaglandin E_1 (misoprostol)	**tPROM**	term premature rupture of the membranes
PGE_2	prostaglandin E_2 (dinoprostone)		
$PGF_2\alpha$	Prostaglandin $F_2\alpha$	**TRAP sequence**	twin reversed arterial perfusion sequence
PIH	pregnancy-induced hypertension		
PKU	phenylketonuria	**TSH**	thyroid stimulating hormone
po	orally	**TTP**	thrombotic thrombocytopenic purpura
PPD	purified protein derivative		
PPH	postpartum hemorrhage	**TTTS**	twin-to-twin transfusion syndrome
pPROM	preterm premature rupture of membranes		
		UA C&S	urine culture and sensitivity
PPS	postpartum sterilization	**UFH**	unfractionated heparin
PRBC	packed red blood cells	**UTI**	urinary tract infection
PROM	premature rupture of membranes	**V/Q scan**	ventilation/perfusion scan
PT	prothrombin time	**VAS**	vibroacoustic stimulation
PTT	partial thromboplastin time	**VBAC**	vaginal birth after cesarean
PTU	propylthiouracil	**VDRL**	venereal disease research laboratory
PUBS	percutaneous umbilical blood sampling	**VL**	viral load
		VTE	venous thromboembolic events
q8h	every eight hours	**WCC**	white cell count

SECTION 1
Preventive Health

Levels of evidence

The levels of evidence used in this book are those recommended by the U.S. Preventive Services Task Force, an independent panel of experts responsible for developing evidence-based recommendations for primary care and prevention, in 2007 (http://www.ahrq.gov/clinic/uspstmeth.htm):

Level I: Evidence obtained from at least one properly designed randomized controlled trial.
Level II: Evidence obtained from controlled trials without randomization or cohort / case-controlled studies that include a comparison group.
Level III: Evidence from uncontrolled descriptive studies (including case series) or opinions of respected authorities or expert committees.
Level IV: Evidence from uncontrolled descriptive studies (including case series) or opinions of respected authorities or expert committees.

1 Abnormal Pap Smear

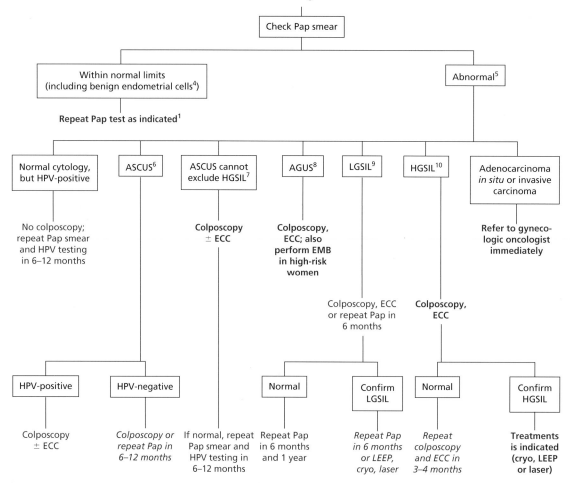

Determine screening frequency

A number of factors influence screening frequency:
- A woman's age[1]
- Prior hysterectomy[2]
- Risk factors for cervical/vaginal cancer[3]

Check Pap smear

Within normal limits (including benign endometrial cells[4])

Abnormal[5]

Repeat Pap test as indicated[1]

Normal cytology, but HPV-positive

ASCUS[6]

ASCUS cannot exclude HGSIL[7]

AGUS[8]

LGSIL[9]

HGSIL[10]

Adenocarcinoma *in situ* or invasive carcinoma

No colposcopy; repeat Pap smear and HPV testing in 6–12 months

Colposcopy ± ECC

Colposcopy, ECC; also perform EMB in high-risk women

Refer to gynecologic oncologist immediately

Colposcopy, ECC or repeat Pap in 6 months

Colposcopy, ECC

HPV-positive

HPV-negative

Normal

Confirm LGSIL

Normal

Confirm HGSIL

Colposcopy ± ECC

Colposcopy or repeat Pap in 6–12 months

If normal, repeat Pap smear and HPV testing in 6–12 months

Repeat Pap in 6 months and 1 year

Repeat Pap in 6 months or LEEP, cryo, laser

Repeat colposcopy and ECC in 3–4 months

Treatments is indicated (cryo, LEEP or laser)

1. Guidelines for screening frequency are based on 2004 recommendations by the American Cancer Society for detection of cervical cancer. Pap tests should be performed for women annually, starting within 3 years of first vaginal intercourse and no later than age 21. For women over 30 years of age who have had three sequential normal Pap tests, screening may be done every 2–3 years. Women over 70 years of age with ≥3 sequential normal

Obstetric Clinical Algorithms: Management and Evidence. By © E.R. Norwitz, M. Belfort, G.R. Saade and H. Miller.
Published 2010 Blackwell Publishing.

Pap tests and no abnormal tests in the last 10 years may stop screening altogether. Women with a history of cervical cancer or other risk factors should continue screening.

2. Women who have had a total hysterectomy may choose to stop screening altogether, unless the surgery was performed for cancer or precancerous lesions in which case vaginal vault smears are indicated. Women who have had a supracervical hysterectomy (and therefore still have their cervix in place) should continue to follow the guidelines for Pap testing outlined above.

3. Women who have risk factors for cervical/vaginal cancer (such as a history of *in utero* diethylstilbestrol (DES) exposure, HIV, women who are immune compromised or those on chronic steroids) should be screened annually.

4. Finding of benign endometrial cells occurs in 10% of Pap smears from premenopausal women and 0.01–0.5% of postmenopausal women. The incidence varies throughout the menstrual cycle and with the use of oral contraceptives or hormone replacement therapy. Of note, the presence of benign endometrial cells in a postmenopausal woman should raise concerns about endometrial cancer, especially if associated with postmenopausal vaginal bleeding. All such women should have an endometrial biopsy (EMB).

5. Women should always be informed of an abnormal Pap result by their physician or another healthcare professional who can answer basic questions and allay anxiety. Verbal notification should be followed with written information and clear recommendations for follow-up. Additionally, if there is evidence of infection along with cellular abnormalities, the infection should be treated.

6. Controversy exists as to whether all women with atypical squamous cells of undetermined significance (ASCUS) smears should be referred for colposcopy. Clinicians should consider risk factors and reliability of patient follow-up in determining whether or not to proceed directly to colposcopy. Women who test positive for high-risk (oncogenic) HPV serotypes (including 16, 18, 31) should be referred immediately for colposcopy. An endocervical curettage (ECC) is indicated if the colposcopy cannot adequately visualize the transformation zone; ECC is contraindicated in pregnancy. If a postmenopausal woman has an ASCUS Pap test and is not on hormone replacement therapy, consider treating her for 6 weeks with vaginal estrogen and repeating the Pap test in 3–4 months. If ASCUS cytology persists, she should be referred for colposcopy and ECC.

7. This category includes 5–10% of all ASCUS smears. The likelihood that this actually represents low-grade squamous intraepithelial lesions (LGSIL) or high-grade squamous intraepithelial lesions (HGSIL) is 10–20%. As such, all such women should be referred for colposcopy. All lesions should be biopsied. If no lesions are evident on colposcopy, then an ECC should be performed.

8. Abnormal glandular cells of undetermined significance (AGUS) warrants an aggressive investigation and close follow-up. All such women should have colposcopy with ECC. Although many of all these patients will have a normal exam on colposcopy, 20–60% will have a significant lesion. In addition, an EMB should be performed in women with AGUS who are >35 years of age with abnormal vaginal bleeding, are morbidly obese, have oligomenorrhea or have clinical results suggesting endometrial cancer. Normal exams should be followed up with Pap smears every 6 months for 2 years.

9. Approximately 60% of LGSIL will regress spontaneously without treatment. Such lesions can be followed by either repeat Pap test in 6 months or colposcopy and ECC. Recent studies suggest a high rate of loss to follow-up and a small risk of delaying diagnosis of cancer and therefore recommend colposcopy/direct biopsy/ECC unless special circumstances exist (such as pregnancy or adolescence). Treatment will depend on the histologic lesion. Cervical intraepithelial neoplasia 1 (CIN 1) can be managed expectantly; CIN 2 and 3 (in the absence of pregnancy) should be managed by excision (loop electrosurgical excision procedure (LEEP)) or ablation (cryotherapy, laser). After treatment, Pap smears should be performed every 3–4 months for a minimum of 1 year. The goal of colposcopy in pregnancy is to exclude invasive cancer.

10. High-grade squamous intraepithelial lesions can progress to invasive cervical cancer. Colposcopy and ECC are therefore recommended in all such women. Treatment is indicated if HGSIL is confirmed. After treatment, Pap smears should be performed every 3 months for 1 year. If the patient is young, nulliparous, and likely to follow up, one can consider q 3–4 monthly Pap smears, with colposcopy/ECC and treatment if HGSIL is persistent.

2 Immunization

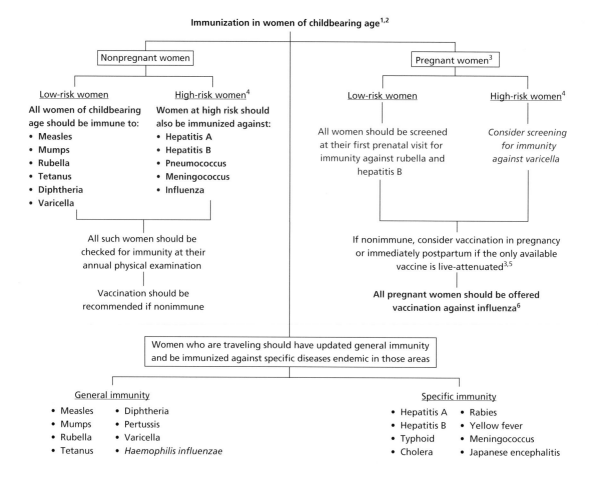

Immunization in women of childbearing age[1,2]

Nonpregnant women

Low-risk women

All women of childbearing age should be immune to:
• **Measles**
• **Mumps**
• **Rubella**
• **Tetanus**
• **Diphtheria**
• **Varicella**

High-risk women[4]

Women at high risk should also be immunized against:
• **Hepatitis A**
• **Hepatitis B**
• **Pneumococcus**
• **Meningococcus**
• **Influenza**

All such women should be checked for immunity at their annual physical examination

Vaccination should be recommended if nonimmune

Pregnant women[3]

Low-risk women

All women should be screened at their first prenatal visit for immunity against rubella and hepatitis B

High-risk women[4]

Consider screening for immunity against varicella

If nonimmune, consider vaccination in pregnancy or immediately postpartum if the only available vaccine is live-attenuated[3,5]

All pregnant women should be offered vaccination against influenza[6]

Women who are traveling should have updated general immunity and be immunized against specific diseases endemic in those areas

General immunity
• Measles   • Diphtheria
• Mumps   • Pertussis
• Rubella   • Varicella
• Tetanus   • *Haemophilis influenzae*

Specific immunity
• Hepatitis A   • Rabies
• Hepatitis B   • Yellow fever
• Typhoid   • Meningococcus
• Cholera   • Japanese encephalitis

Obstetric Clinical Algorithms: Management and Evidence. By © E.R. Norwitz, M. Belfort, G.R. Saade and H. Miller.
Published 2010 Blackwell Publishing.

1. Immunization can be active (vaccines, toxoid) or passive (immunoglobulin, antiserum/antitoxin). In *active immunity*, the immune response is induced by wild infection or vaccination, which is generally robust and long-lasting. As such, subsequent exposure to the vaccine-preventable infection will result in release of antibodies and prevention of illness. In *passive immunity*, antibodies are acquired passively through maternal transfer across the placenta or breast milk or through receipt of exogenous immunoglobulins. Protection is temporary and fades within a few weeks to months. The immune system of the recipient is therefore not programmed, and subsequent exposure to vaccine-preventable infections can lead to active infection.

2. Vaccination works by inducing antibodies in recipients that protect them against infection after future exposure to specific disease-causing microbes. The level of protection varies according to the strength and durability of the immune response induced by the vaccine as well as the virulence, prevalence, and ease of transmission of the infection itself. Vaccination programs may have different goals: (i) to protect at-risk individuals (e.g. meningococcal disease), (ii) to establish control by minimizing the overall prevalence of the infection (e.g. measles, varicella) or (iii) to attain global elimination of an infection (e.g. neonatal tetanus, polio).

3. Vaccination in pregnancy is of concern because of the increased vulnerability of the fetus. Inactivated vaccines are approved for use in pregnancy. However, live-attenuated vaccines (including rubella, MMR, varicella) are not recommended for pregnant women despite the fact that no cases of congenital anomalies have ever been documented. Exceptions include yellow fever and polio, which are live-attenuated vaccines but can be given to pregnant women when traveling to high-prevalence areas. In addition, women should be advised not to get pregnant within 1 month of receiving a live-attenuated vaccine. Vaccines considered safe in pregnancy include tetanus, diphtheria, hepatitis B, and influenza. Tetanus immunization during pregnancy is a common strategy used in the developing world to combat neonatal tetanus.

4. Risk factors for specific vaccine preventable illnesses include:
- illicit drug users (hepatitis A and B, tetanus)
- men who have sex with men (hepatitis A)
- >1 sexual partner in the past 6 months (hepatitis A, human papillomavirus)
- travel to or immigration from areas where infection is endemic (hepatitis A and B, measles, meningococcus, rubella, tetanus, varicella)
- healthcare workers (hepatitis B, influenza, varicella)
- nursing home residents (meningococcus, pneumococcus, varicella)
- a history of sexually transmitted infections (hepatitis B)
- chronic medical conditions such as diabetes, asthma, HIV, chronic liver disease, chronic renal disease, and immunosuppression (hepatitis A, influenza, pneumococcus)
- ≥50 years of age (influenza)
- adults who have had their spleens removed (meningococcus, pneumococcus)
- accidental or intentional puncture wounds (tetanus).

5. One of the current controversies about vaccination in pregnancy is whether vaccines containing thimerosal pose a risk to the fetus. Thimerosal is a mercury-containing preservative used in vaccines since the 1930s. Although it is not clear what the source is, some infants who have received vaccines within the first 6 months of life have been shown to have cumulative levels of mercury that exceed US Environmental Protection Agency-recommended guidelines. In response to these reports, in 1999, the American Academy of Pediatrics (AAP) and various US governmental agencies advocated reducing or eliminating thimerosal in childhood vaccines. While many childhood vaccines in use today are preservative free, adult versions may not be. Because some research (but not all) suggests that thimerosal exposure in infants could be related to neurodevelopmental problems, it is prudent to avoid thimerosal-containing vaccines in pregnancy. The following adult vaccines are thimerosal free: Tdap (but not Td), Recombivax hepatitis B vaccine (but not Engerix-B), and some influenza vaccines (Fluzone with no thimerosal).

6. Immunization with the trivalent inactivated influenza vaccine (TIV) is recommended during influenza season (November through March in the northern hemisphere) for all pregnant women, both high and low risk, at any point in the pregnancy. The newer influenza vaccine, the live-attenuated viral influenza vaccine (LAIV), is contraindicated in pregnancy.

3 Preconception Care

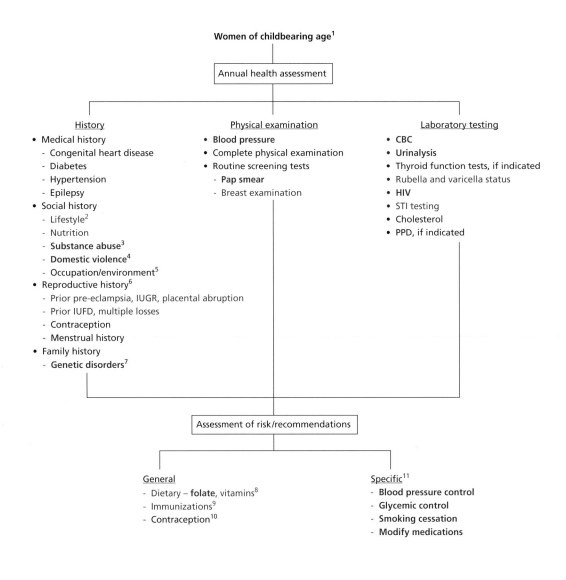

Women of childbearing age[1]

Annual health assessment

History
- Medical history
  - Congenital heart disease
  - Diabetes
  - Hypertension
  - Epilepsy
- Social history
  - Lifestyle[2]
  - Nutrition
  - **Substance abuse[3]**
  - **Domestic violence[4]**
  - **Occupation/environment[5]**
- Reproductive history[6]
  - Prior pre-eclampsia, IUGR, placental abruption
  - Prior IUFD, multiple losses
  - Contraception
  - Menstrual history
- Family history
  - **Genetic disorders[7]**

Physical examination
- **Blood pressure**
- Complete physical examination
- Routine screening tests
  - **Pap smear**
  - Breast examination

Laboratory testing
- **CBC**
- **Urinalysis**
- Thyroid function tests, if indicated
- Rubella and varicella status
- **HIV**
- STI testing
- Cholesterol
- PPD, if indicated

Assessment of risk/recommendations

General
- Dietary – **folate**, vitamins[8]
- Immunizations[9]
- Contraception[10]

Specific[11]
- **Blood pressure control**
- **Glycemic control**
- **Smoking cessation**
- **Modify medications**

Obstetric Clinical Algorithms: Management and Evidence. By © E.R. Norwitz, M. Belfort, G.R. Saade and H. Miller.
Published 2010 Blackwell Publishing.

1. Fetal organogenesis occurs before most women are aware that they are pregnant. As such, the ideal time for addressing primary prevention of reproductive health risks is in the preconception period. Since approximately half of all pregnancies in the United States are unplanned, all women of reproductive age should be considered candidates for discussion of these issues.

2. Discuss social, financial and psychological issues in preparation for pregnancy.

3. Maternal alcohol use is the leading known cause of mental retardation, and is the leading preventable cause of birth defects in the Western world. An accurate drinking history, taken with a tool that employs screening questions (such as the CAGE questionnaire), is critical. Effects of alcohol may be compounded with abuse of other drugs. Cigarette smoking, cocaine, and other drug use should be included in the history. Provide education, brief intervention, contraceptive counseling, and referral for treatment as necessary.

4. Screen for domestic violence. Be aware of available state and local resources available and state laws regarding reporting. Risk increases with pregnancy. Domestic violence is not isolated to any risk group other than pregnancy; it cuts across socio-economic and ethnic lines.

5. Take an occupational history that will allow assessment of workplace risks to pregnancy. Elicit information about any exposures to hazardous materials or biologic hazards (HIV, CMV, toxoplasmosis) and use of safety equipment.

6. Counsel patients with history of pre-eclampsia, placental abruption, unexplained fetal death, or severe IUGR about the potential risk of recurrence. The use of low-dose aspirin, calcium supplementation, and/or anticoagulation for women with documented inherited thrombophilias to prevent adverse pregnancy outcome is controversial, and cannot be routinely recommended.

7. Personal and family histories should be examined for evidence of genetic diseases. Screening of carriers are available for some autosomal recessive conditions such as Tay–Sachs, Canavan disease, sickle cell disease, and the thalassemias. Consider referrals for further genetic counseling if patients are at high risk. ACOG currently requires that all couples be offered prenatal testing for cystic fibrosis.

8. Emphasize the importance of nutrition. Assess appropriateness of patient's weight for height, special diets and nutrition patterns such as vegetarianism, fasting, pica, bulimia, and vitamin supplementation. Recommend folic acid supplementation as necessary: 0.4 mg per day for all, 4.0 mg per day if the woman has had a child with a neural tube defect or is on anticonvulsant medications (especially valproic acid). Counsel avoidance of oversupplementation (such as vitamin A). Review recommendations on dietary fish ($<$12 ounces per week of cooked fish) to reduce mercury intake, and steps for prevention of listeriosis (avoiding raw or undercooked meat/fish, unpasteurized milk and soft cheeses, unwashed fruit and vegetables) and toxoplasmosis (exposure to cat feces).

9. An immunization history should be obtained that addresses vaccination. Women should be tested for immunity to rubella and vaccinated if not immune. Women without a history of chickenpox (varicella) should be tested and offered vaccination. Hepatitis B vaccination should be offered to all women at high-risk, and screening for other sexually transmitted infections should be offered. The CDC recommends that pregnancy be delayed for at least 1 month after MMR vaccination.

10. Discuss birth spacing and choices of contraception.

11. Effects of the pregnancy on any medical conditions for both mother and fetus should be discussed. Medications should be reviewed, and patients counseled regarding alternatives that may be safer in pregnancy. Close communication with the patient's primary care and subspecialty physicians should always be maintained.

4 Prenatal Care[1]

Initial prenatal visit

- Take a detailed history and physical examination
- Send routine prenatal laboratory tests[2]

Low-risk pregnancy

High-risk pregnancy[3]

Issues that should be addressed routinely:

- **Folic acid supplementation** (1 mg daily for all reproductive age women) to prevent neural tube defect
- Identify and treat existing sexually transmitted infections, diabetes, thyroid disease, obesity, HIV, hepatitis B
- Identify maternal phenylketonuria (PKU)
- **Discontinue teratogenic drugs (such as coumadin, vitamin A)**
- **Counsel on risks of smoking, alcohol, and illicit drug use**
- Counsel about appropriate use of seatbelts and airbags
- *Reassure about safety of sexual intercourse, moderate exercise*
- **Screen for domestic violence and depression**
- Review symptoms/signs of complications (e.g. preterm birth)
- **Check rubella immunity status**
- Ask about chickenpox (√ varicella immunity status if unknown)
- Counsel about toxoplasmosis prevention
- **Counsel about influenza vaccination in pregnancy**
- Counsel about food safety, multivitamins
- Encourage breastfeeding

Regular follow-up prenatal visits[4]

Routine testing for all low-risk pregnancies
- Weight/Body Mass Index (BMI in kg/m^2) at each prenatal visit
- **BP and urine dipstix at each prenatal visit[5]**
- **UA C&S q trimester to exclude asymptomatic bacteriuria and urinary tract infection (UTI)**
- 1st trimester risk assessment for fetal aneuploidy[6]
- *Serum analyte ("quad") screen for fetal aneuploidy at 15–20 weeks[6]*
- MS-AFP for neural tube defect at 15–20 weeks[6]
- PPD (to screen for TB exposure) in 2nd trimester
- **1-hour GLT screening for gestational diabetes (GDM) at 24–28 weeks[7]**
- **GBS perineal culture at 35–36 weeks[8]**

- Address issues as for low-risk pregnancies (opposite)
- Schedule follow-up visits based on individual risk factors
- Individualize prenatal testing based on risk factors

Maternal tests

- Hemoglobin electrophoresis (for sickle cell trait in African-Americans; for β-thalassemia in Mediterranean/Italians)
- Genetics testing for α-thalassemia in Mediterranean/Italians (esp. if anemia unresponsive to iron supplementation)
- **Urine toxicology screen (for women with a history of illicit drug use)**
- Chest x-ray if PPD positive
- Smoking cessation counseling
- Baseline renal/liver function tests, 24-hour urinalysis in high-risk patients[5]
- Early GLT screening for GDM at 16–20 weeks in high-risk patients[7]
- **3-hour GTT to confirm diagnosis of GDM in women with a positive GLT[7]**
- Cervical length and fetal fibronectin in women at risk of preterm birth[9]
- **UA C&S q month in women at high risk for UTI (diabetes, sickle cell trait, history of recurrent UTI, HIV)**
- Maternal EKG, echo, cardiology consultation in women at risk

Fetal tests

- Early dating ultrasound to confirm gestational age, exclude multiple pregnancy
- Genetic counseling in high-risk women (e.g. AMA, personal or family history of an inherited disorder, abnormal aneuploidy screening test, CF carrier)
- **Genetic amniocentesis/CVS to exclude fetal aneuploidy[6]**
- Fetal anatomic survey (level II ultrasound) at 18–20 weeks
- Fetal echo at 20–22 weeks to diagnose cardiac anomaly in women at high risk
- **Serial ultrasounds for fetal growth q 3–4 weeks after 24 weeks in pregnancies at risk for IUGR or macrosomia**
- Fetal testing q week after 32 weeks in high-risk women (e.g. diabetes, AMA, chronic hypertension)
- **Amniocentesis at 36–38 weeks for fetal lung maturity testing**

Obstetric Clinical Algorithms: Management and Evidence. By © E.R. Norwitz, M. Belfort, G.R. Saade and H. Miller.
Published 2010 Blackwell Publishing.

1. The goal of prenatal care is to promote the health and well-being of the pregnant woman, fetus, infant, and family up to 1 year after birth. To achieve these aims, prenatal care must be available and accessible. The three major components are: (i) early and continuing risk assessment, including preconception assessment; (ii) continued health promotion; and (iii) both medical and psychosocial assessment and intervention.

2. Routine prenatal tests that should be sent in all pregnant women include complete blood count (CBC), blood group type and screen ($\sqrt{}$ Rh status), rubella serology, HIV, hepatitis B, syphilis serology (VDRL/RPR), Pap smear, cystic fibrosis (CF) carrier status, chlamydia/gonorrhea cultures, and urine culture and sensitivity (UA C&S).

3. Approximately 20% (1 in 5) of pregnancies are considered high risk. Risk factors for adverse pregnancy outcome may exist prior to pregnancy or develop during pregnancy or even during labor (examples are listed below, although this list should not be regarded as comprehensive).

4. The frequency and timing of prenatal visits will vary depending on the risk status of the pregnant woman and her fetus. In low-risk women, prenatal visits are typically recommended q 4 weeks to 28 weeks, q 2 weeks to 36 weeks, and then weekly until delivery.

5. See Chapter 12 (Pre-eclampsia)

6. See Chapter 50 (Prenatal diagnosis)

7. See Chapter 10 (Gestational diabetes)

8. See Chapter 24 (GBS)

9. See Chapter 52 (Screening for preterm birth)

High-Risk Pregnancies

Maternal factors

- Pre-existing medical conditions (diabetes, chronic hypertension, cardiac disease, renal disease, pulmonary disease)
- Pre-eclampsia

- Gestational diabetes
- Morbid obesity
- Extremes of maternal age
- Active venous thromboembolic disease

- Poor obstetric history (prior preterm birth, preterm PROM, stillbirth, IUGR, placental abruption, pre-eclampsia, recurrent miscarriage)

Fetal factors

- Fetal structural or chromosomal anomaly
- History of a prior baby with a structural or chromosomal anomaly
- Family history of a genetic syndrome

- Toxic exposure (to environmental toxins, medications, illicit drugs)
- IUGR
- Fetal macrosomia

- Multiple pregnancy (esp. if monochorionic)
- Isoimmunization
- Intra-amniotic infection (chorioamnionitis)
- Nonreassuring fetal testing

Uteroplacental factors

- Preterm premature rupture of membranes
- Unexplained oligohydramnios
- Large uterine fibroids (esp. if submucosal)
- Prior cervical insufficiency

- Prior uterine surgery (especially prior "classic" hysterotomy)
- Placental abruption
- Placenta previa

- Uterine anomaly (didelphys, septate)
- Abnormal placentation (placenta accreta, increta or percreta)
- Vasa previa

SECTION 2
Maternal Disorders

Levels of evidence

The levels of evidence used in this book are those recommended by the U.S. Preventive Services Task Force, an independent panel of experts responsible for developing evidence-based recommendations for primary care and prevention, in 2007 (http://www.ahrq.gov/clinic/uspstmeth.htm):

Level I: Evidence obtained from at least one properly designed randomized controlled trial.
Level II: Evidence obtained from controlled trials without randomization or cohort / case-controlled studies that include a comparison group.
Level III: Evidence from uncontrolled descriptive studies (including case series) or opinions of respected authorities or expert committees.
Level IV: Evidence from uncontrolled descriptive studies (including case series) or opinions of respected authorities or expert committees.

5 Antiphospholipid Antibody Syndrome

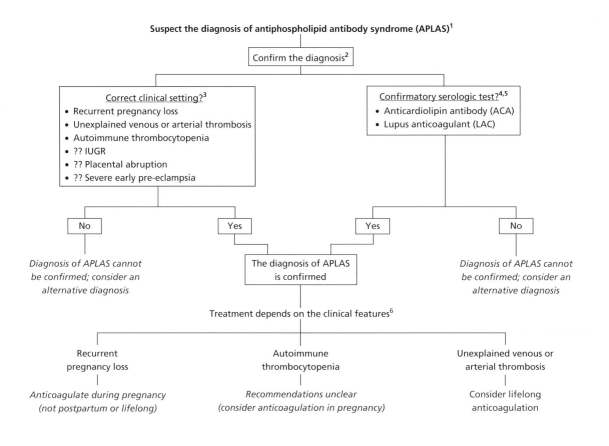

Suspect the diagnosis of antiphospholipid antibody syndrome (APLAS)[1]

Confirm the diagnosis[2]

Correct clinical setting?[3]
- Recurrent pregnancy loss
- Unexplained venous or arterial thrombosis
- Autoimmune thrombocytopenia
- ?? IUGR
- ?? Placental abruption
- ?? Severe early pre-eclampsia

Confirmatory serologic test?[4,5]
- Anticardiolipin antibody (ACA)
- Lupus anticoagulant (LAC)

No — *Diagnosis of APLAS cannot be confirmed; consider an alternative diagnosis*

Yes — The diagnosis of APLAS is confirmed

Yes — The diagnosis of APLAS is confirmed

No — *Diagnosis of APLAS cannot be confirmed; consider an alternative diagnosis*

Treatment depends on the clinical features[6]

Recurrent pregnancy loss — *Anticoagulate during pregnancy (not postpartum or lifelong)*

Autoimmune thrombocytopenia — *Recommendations unclear (consider anticoagulation in pregnancy)*

Unexplained venous or arterial thrombosis — Consider lifelong anticoagulation

1. Antiphospholipid antibody syndrome (APLAS) is an autoimmune disease characterized by the presence in the maternal circulation of one or more autoantibodies against membrane phospholipid as well as one or more specific clinical syndromes. It is an acquired rather than inherited condition. As such, it cannot explain a family history of venous thromboembolic events (VTE). A significant family history of VTE should prompt testing to exclude inherited thrombophilias, including factor V Leiden mutation, prothrombin gene mutation, and protein S, protein C, and antithrombin deficiency.

2. The diagnosis of APLAS requires two distinct elements: (i) the correct clinical setting, and (ii) confirmatory serologic testing. Approximately 2–4% of healthy pregnant women will have circulating antiphospholipid antibodies in the absence of any clinical symptoms. As such, routine screening for these antibodies in all pregnant women is strongly discouraged.

3. Clinical manifestations of APLAS include: (1) recurrent pregnancy loss (defined as ≥3 unexplained first-trimester pregnancy losses or ≥1 unexplained second-trimester pregnancy loss); (2) unexplained thrombosis (venous, arterial,

Obstetric Clinical Algorithms: Management and Evidence. By © E.R. Norwitz, M. Belfort, G.R. Saade and H. Miller.
Published 2010 Blackwell Publishing.

cerebrovascular accident or myocardial infarction); and/or (3) autoimmune thrombocytopenia (platelets <100,000/mm^3). Some consensus opinions include such clinical conditions as unexplained intrauterine fetal growth restriction (IUGR), placental abruption, and severe early pre-eclampsia, but this remains controversial.

4. At least one of two serologic tests confirming the presence of circulating antiphospholipid antibodies is required to make the diagnosis of APLAS.

- Lupus anticoagulant (LAC) is an unidentified antiphospholipid antibody (or antibodies) that causes prolongation of phospholipid-dependent coagulation tests *in vitro* by binding to the prothrombin–activator complex. Examples of tests that can confirm the presence of LAC include the activated PTT test, dilute Russel viper venom test, kaolin clotting time, and recalcification time. *In vivo*, however, LAC causes thrombosis. LAC results are reported as present or absent (no titers are given). The term LAC is a misnomer: it is not specific to lupus (SLE) and it acts *in vivo* as a procoagulant and not an anticoagulant.
- Antibodies against specific phospholipids as measured by ELISA. These high-avidity IgG antibodies have anticoagulant activity *in vitro* but procoagulant activity *in vivo*. The most commonly used ELISA test is anticardiolipin antibody (ACA). Cardiolipin is a negatively charged phospholipid isolated from ox heart. ACA ELISA is at best semi-quantitative. Results have traditionally been reported as low, medium or high titers. More recently, standardization of the phospholipid extract has allowed for standard units to be developed (GPL units for IgG, MPL units for IgM). ACA IgM alone, IgA alone, and/or low-positive IgG may be a nonspecific (incidental) finding since they are present in 2–4% of asymptomatic pregnant women. As such, moderate-to-high levels of ACA IgG (>40 GPL units) are required to make the diagnosis of APLAS. Moreover, since such antibodies may be nonspecific, most consensus statements require two positive tests at least 8 weeks apart to confirm the diagnosis.

5. A number of additional antiphospholipid antibodies are described, including antiphosphatidylserine, antiphosphatidylethanolamine, antiphosphatidylcholine, anti-Ro,

and anti-La, but these are not sufficient to make the diagnosis. A false-positive test for syphilis (defined as a positive rapid plasma reagin (RPR) or Venereal Disease Research Laboratory (VDRL) test, but negative definitive test for syphilis) is another common finding in women with APLAS, but is nonspecific and is not sufficient to confirm the diagnosis. Antinuclear antibodies (ANA) are not antiphospholipid antibodies, and suggest the diagnosis of SLE and not APLAS.

6. Treatment for APLAS depends on the clinical features.

- For women with thrombosis (such as stroke or pulmonary embolism), *therapeutic* anticoagulation is indicated with either unfractionated heparin (UFH) or low molecular weight heparin (LMWH) during pregnancy followed by oral anticoagulation (coumadin) postpartum because of a 5–15% risk of recurrence. In pregnancy, regular blood tests are required 4 hours after administration of the drug to ensure that anticoagulation is therapeutic: the PTT should be 1.5- to 2.5-fold normal and anti-Xa activity levels should be 0.6–1.0 U/mL. Side-effects include hemorrhage, thrombocytopenia, and osteopenia and fractures. Such women may need lifelong treatment.
- For women with recurrent pregnancy loss, treatment should include *prophylactic* UFH (5000–10,000 units sc bid) or LMWH (enoxaparin (Lovenox) 30–40 mg sc daily or dalteparin (Fragmin) 2500–5000 U sc daily) starting in the first trimester of pregnancy. Although prophylactic dosing does not change PTT, it will increase anti-Xa activity to 0.1–0.2 U/mL. However, it is not necessary to follow serial anti-Xa activity in such patients. The goal of this treatment is to prevent pregnancy loss and to prevent VTE, which is possible in women with APLAS in pregnancy even if they have not had a VTE in the past. Therefore, anticoagulation should be administered throughout pregnancy and (possibly) for 6–12 weeks after delivery.
- For women with autoimmune thrombocytopenia or a history of severe pre-eclampsia, IUGR or placental abruption, the optimal treatment is unknown. Consider treating as for recurrent pregnancy loss. Postpartum anticoagulation is probably not necessary.

6 Asthma

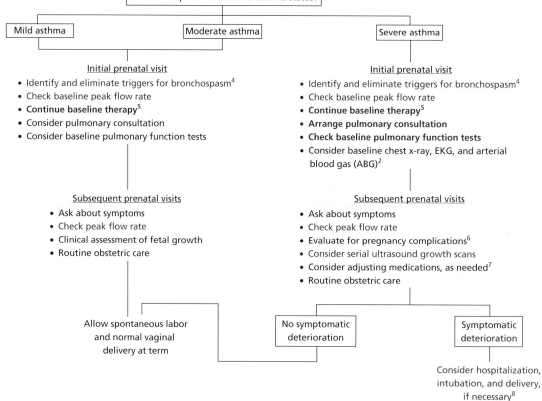

Confirm the diagnosis of asthma

- Take a detailed history, perform a physical examination, and perform relevant pulmonary tests[1]
- Be aware of the normal physiologic changes in the respiratory system during pregnancy[2]
- Consider differential diagnosis[3]

What is the patient's baseline asthma status?

| Mild asthma | Moderate asthma | Severe asthma |

Initial prenatal visit

- Identify and eliminate triggers for bronchospasm[4]
- Check baseline peak flow rate
- **Continue baseline therapy[5]**
- Consider pulmonary consultation
- Consider baseline pulmonary function tests

Initial prenatal visit

- Identify and eliminate triggers for bronchospasm[4]
- Check baseline peak flow rate
- **Continue baseline therapy[5]**
- **Arrange pulmonary consultation**
- **Check baseline pulmonary function tests**
- Consider baseline chest x-ray, EKG, and arterial blood gas (ABG)[2]

Subsequent prenatal visits

- Ask about symptoms
- Check peak flow rate
- Clinical assessment of fetal growth
- Routine obstetric care

Subsequent prenatal visits

- Ask about symptoms
- Check peak flow rate
- Evaluate for pregnancy complications[6]
- Consider serial ultrasound growth scans
- Consider adjusting medications, as needed[7]
- Routine obstetric care

Allow spontaneous labor and normal vaginal delivery at term

No symptomatic deterioration

Symptomatic deterioration

Consider hospitalization, intubation, and delivery, if necessary[8]

Obstetric Clinical Algorithms: Management and Evidence. By © E.R. Norwitz, M. Belfort, G.R. Saade and H. Miller.
Published 2010 Blackwell Publishing.

1. Asthma is a chronic inflammatory disorder of the airways characterized by intermittent episodes of reversible bronchospasm. The "classic" signs and symptoms of asthma are intermittent dyspnea, cough, and wheezing. Pulmonary function tests that are most helpful in diagnosing asthma are peak expiratory flow rate (PEFR), spirometry (which includes measurement of forced expiratory volume in one second (FEV1) and forced vital capacity (FVC)), and bronchoprovocation testing (such as with a metacholine or exercise challenge). Findings consistent with asthma include a variability of >20% in PEFR, a reduction in FEV1 and FEV1/FVC ratio on spirometry, an increase in FEV1 of more than 15% from the baseline following administration of 2–4 puffs of a bronchodilator, and heightened sensitivity to bronchoprovocation. Asthma complicates 1–4% of all pregnancies. Pregnancy has a variable effect on asthma (25% improve, 25% worsen, 50% are unchanged). In general, women with mild, well-controlled asthma tolerate pregnancy well. Women with severe asthma are at risk of symptomatic deterioration.

2. Respiratory adaptations during pregnancy are designed to optimize maternal and fetal oxygenation, and to facilitate transfer of CO_2 waste from the fetus to the mother. The mechanics of respiration change with pregnancy. The ribs flare outward and the level of the diaphragm rises 4 cm. During pregnancy, tidal volume increases by 200 mL (40%), resulting in a 100–200 mL (5%) increase in vital capacity and a 200 mL (20%) decrease in the residual volume, thereby leaving less air in the lungs at the end of expiration. The respiratory rate does not change. The end result is an increase in minute ventilation and a drop in arterial PCO_2. Arterial PO_2 is essentially unchanged. A compensatory decrease in bicarbonate enables the pH to remain unchanged. Pregnancy thus represents a state of *compensated respiratory alkalosis*.

	pH	PO_2 (mmHg)	PCO_2 (mmHg)
Nonpregnant	7.40	93–100	35–40
Pregnant	7.40	100–105	28–30

3. The differential diagnosis of asthma includes pneumonia, pulmonary embolism, pneumothorax, congestive cardiac failure, pericarditis, pulmonary edema, and rib fracture.

4. Characteristic triggers for asthma include exercise, cold air, and exposure to allergens. Exercise-triggered symptoms typically develop 10–15 min after exertion and are more intense when the inhaled air is cold. Allergens that typically trigger asthma symptoms include dust, molds, furred animals, cockroaches, pollens, and other irritant-type exposures (cigarette smoke, strong fumes, airborne chemicals). Viral infections can also trigger asthma symptoms. Influenza vaccination is recommended (see Chapter 2).

5. The principal goals of treatment are to minimize symptoms, normalize pulmonary function, prevent exacerbations, and improve health-related quality of life. Initial treatment for relief of symptoms should be an inhaled short-acting β-agonist used on an as-needed basis rather than at regularly scheduled intervals. The most commonly agent is an albuterol inhaler at a dose of 2–4 puffs as needed every 4–6 hours. If this is not adequate to control symptoms, inhaled glucocorticoids (such as beclometasone dipropionate) should be given by metered dose inhaler (MDI) and should be taken at regular intervals 2–3 times daily.

6. Pregnancy-related complications of severe asthma include intrauterine growth restriction (IUGR), stillbirth, and maternal mortality.

7. A number of alternative therapies are available on an outpatient basis. These include a short course of oral glucocorticoids. A typical regimen is prednisone 0.5 mg per kg bodyweight given orally each day and tapered over a period of 1–2 weeks. This can be given alone or in combination with a leukotriene-modifying agent – such as the leukotriene D4 receptor antagonists zafirlukast (Accolate) and montelukast (Singulair) or the 5-lipoxygenase inhibitor zileuton (Zyflo) – or a slow-release theophylline.

8. See Chapter 71 (Acute asthma exacerbation).

7 Cholestasis of Pregnancy

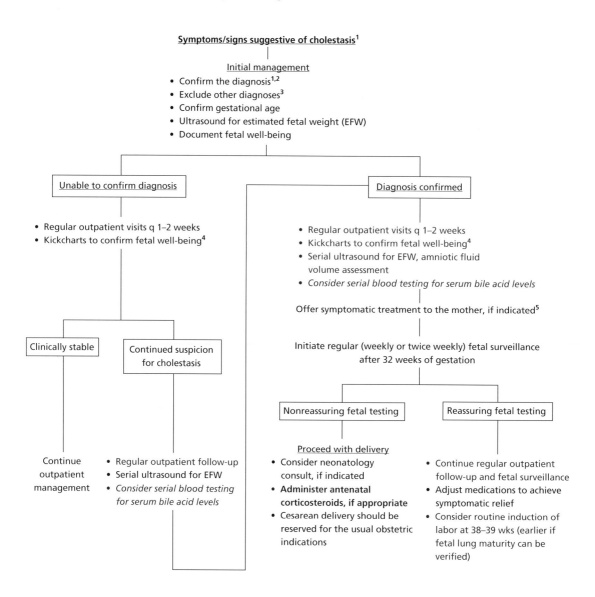

Symptoms/signs suggestive of cholestasis[1]

Initial management
- Confirm the diagnosis[1,2]
- Exclude other diagnoses[3]
- Confirm gestational age
- Ultrasound for estimated fetal weight (EFW)
- Document fetal well-being

Unable to confirm diagnosis

- Regular outpatient visits q 1–2 weeks
- Kickcharts to confirm fetal well-being[4]

Clinically stable

Continued suspicion for cholestasis

Continue outpatient management

- Regular outpatient follow-up
- Serial ultrasound for EFW
- *Consider serial blood testing for serum bile acid levels*

Diagnosis confirmed

- Regular outpatient visits q 1–2 weeks
- Kickcharts to confirm fetal well-being[4]
- Serial ultrasound for EFW, amniotic fluid volume assessment
- *Consider serial blood testing for serum bile acid levels*

Offer symptomatic treatment to the mother, if indicated[5]

Initiate regular (weekly or twice weekly) fetal surveillance after 32 weeks of gestation

Nonreassuring fetal testing

Proceed with delivery
- Consider neonatology consult, if indicated
- **Administer antenatal corticosteroids, if appropriate**
- Cesarean delivery should be reserved for the usual obstetric indications

Reassuring fetal testing

- Continue regular outpatient follow-up and fetal surveillance
- Adjust medications to achieve symptomatic relief
- Consider routine induction of labor at 38–39 wks (earlier if fetal lung maturity can be verified)

Obstetric Clinical Algorithms: Management and Evidence. By © E.R. Norwitz, M. Belfort, G.R. Saade and H. Miller.
Published 2010 Blackwell Publishing.

1. Cholestasis of pregnancy (also known as "benign" cholestasis of pregnancy) represents a clinical syndrome that results from an inability to adequately metabolize and excrete bile acids during pregnancy. Risk factors for cholestasis include cholestasis in a prior pregnancy (recurrence rate is >90%) and underlying liver, renal, and/or bowel disease.

2. Cholestasis of pregnancy is a <u>clinical/biochemical</u> diagnosis. Patients typically present with complaints of acute onset of severe pruritus in the latter half of pregnancy. Physical examination may reveal jaundice and/or skin excoriations, but is often unremarkable. Laboratory tests may reveal elevations in circulating liver function tests and/or bile acids (especially cholic and chenodeoxycholic acid).

3. The differential diagnosis of cholestasis includes skin allergy, parasitic infections, systemic lupus erythematosus (SLE), syphilis, viral/drug-induced hepatitis, pre-eclampsia, metabolic disorders, and gallbladder diseases.

4. Cholestasis of pregnancy is associated with adverse perinatal outcome, including increase perinatal mortality (unexplained stillbirth), premature birth, and meconium passage and aspiration. The association with IUGR is less clear. For these reasons, regular (weekly or twice weekly) fetal surveillance is recommended after 32 weeks of gestation. However, it is not clear whether fetal testing is associated with an improvement in perinatal outcome.

5. In contrast to the effects on the fetus, cholestasis of pregnancy is not associated with adverse maternal outcome. However, the symptoms may be extreme. If so, it may be appropriate to offer the mother symptomatic therapy. The most common agents used are cholestyramine (a foul-tasting resin that binds bile acids in the gastrointestinal system) and ursodeoxycholic acid. Response to such medications may take several weeks and is highly variable. Alternative treatment options that are less well established include ultraviolet light, phenobarbitone, epomediol or *S*-adenosyl-L-methionine.

8 Chronic Hypertension[1]

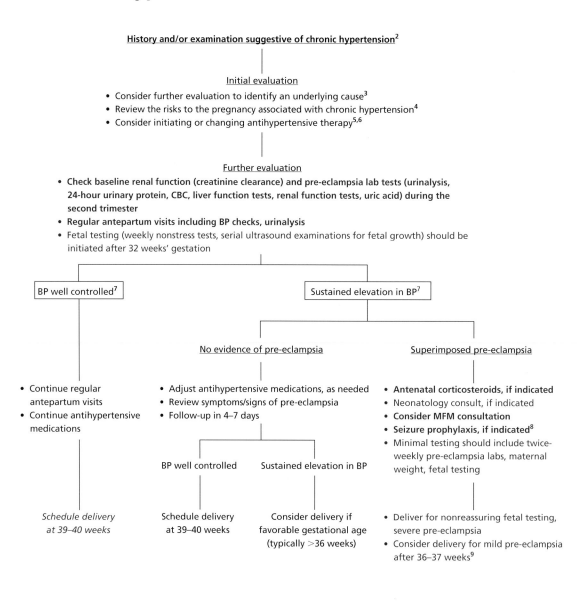

History and/or examination suggestive of chronic hypertension[2]

Initial evaluation
- Consider further evaluation to identify an underlying cause[3]
- Review the risks to the pregnancy associated with chronic hypertension[4]
- Consider initiating or changing antihypertensive therapy[5,6]

Further evaluation
- **Check baseline renal function (creatinine clearance) and pre-eclampsia lab tests (urinalysis, 24-hour urinary protein, CBC, liver function tests, renal function tests, uric acid) during the second trimester**
- **Regular antepartum visits including BP checks, urinalysis**
- Fetal testing (weekly nonstress tests, serial ultrasound examinations for fetal growth) should be initiated after 32 weeks' gestation

BP well controlled[7]

Sustained elevation in BP[7]

No evidence of pre-eclampsia

Superimposed pre-eclampsia

- Continue regular antepartum visits
- Continue antihypertensive medications

- Adjust antihypertensive medications, as needed
- Review symptoms/signs of pre-eclampsia
- Follow-up in 4–7 days

- **Antenatal corticosteroids, if indicated**
- Neonatology consult, if indicated
- **Consider MFM consultation**
- **Seizure prophylaxis, if indicated[8]**
- Minimal testing should include twice-weekly pre-eclampsia labs, maternal weight, fetal testing

BP well controlled

Sustained elevation in BP

Schedule delivery at 39–40 weeks

Schedule delivery at 39–40 weeks

Consider delivery if favorable gestational age (typically >36 weeks)

- Deliver for nonreassuring fetal testing, severe pre-eclampsia
- Consider delivery for mild pre-eclampsia after 36–37 weeks[9]

Obstetric Clinical Algorithms: Management and Evidence. By © E.R. Norwitz, M. Belfort, G.R. Saade and H. Miller.
Published 2010 Blackwell Publishing.

1. Chronic hypertension refers to the presence of hypertension prior to pregnancy, whether or not the patient was on treatment. Given that BP normally decreases in the first and early second trimester of pregnancy, the diagnosis should also be entertained in women with a sustained elevation in BP ≥140/90 prior to 20 weeks' gestation.

2. Most patients with chronic hypertension are asymptomatic. Symptoms such as decreased/increased urine output or hematuria may suggest underlying renal disease.

3. Any women presenting with new-onset chronic hypertension should have a thorough evaluation to identify an underlying cause. Such causes may include renal artery stenosis, chronic renal disease, and an underlying endocrinopathy (such as hyperaldosteronism, Cushing syndrome).

4. Chronic hypertension is associated with an increased risk of superimposed pre-eclampsia, hypertensive crisis and cerebrovascular accident (stroke), uteroplacental insufficiency leading to IUGR, placental abruption, and stillbirth.

5. Treatment of mild hypertension has been shown not to improve pregnancy outcome. As such, it is rarely necessary to initiate antihypertensive therapy in early pregnancy. If a patient is well controlled on medications prior to pregnancy, it is usual to leave her medications unchanged. The exception are the angiotensin-converting enzyme (ACE) inhibitors, which should be discontinued as soon as a positive pregnancy test is attained. These drugs do not increase the risk of structural anomalies, but have been associated with progressive and irreversible renal injury as well as oligohydramnios in the fetus, especially if administered in the second trimester. Drugs of choice include α-methyldopa, β-blockers (labetalol) or calcium channel blockers (nifedipine). Diuretic therapy is generally discouraged in pregnancy.

6. There are only three indications for antihypertensive therapy in the setting of pre-eclampsia: (a) underlying chronic hypertension; (b) to achieve BP control to prevent cerebrovascular accident while effecting delivery; and/or (c) expectant management of severe pre-eclampsia by BP criteria alone less than 32 weeks (Sibai protocol). BP control is important to prevent cerebrovascular accident (usually associated with BP ≥ 170/120 mmHg), but does not affect the natural course of pre-eclampsia.

7. Adequate BP control refers to a sustained sitting BP of <160/110 mmHg.

8. Intravenous magnesium sulfate is the drug of choice and should be given intrapartum and for at least 24 hours postpartum to prevent eclampsia.

9. Delivery is the only effective treatment for pre-eclampsia. It is recommended in women with mild pre-eclampsia once a favorable gestational age has been reached and in all women with severe pre-eclampsia regardless of gestational age (with the exception of severe pre-eclampsia due to proteinuria alone, IUGR remote from term with good fetal testing, or possibly severe pre-eclampsia by BP criteria alone <32 weeks (Sibai protocol)). There is no proven benefit to routine delivery by cesarean. However, the probability of vaginal delivery in a patient with pre-eclampsia remote from term with an unfavorable cervix is only 15–20%. Pre-eclampsia and its complications always resolve following delivery (with the exception of stroke). Diuresis (>4 L/day) is the most accurate clinical indicator of resolution. Fetal prognosis is dependent largely on gestational age at delivery.

9 Deep Vein Thrombosis

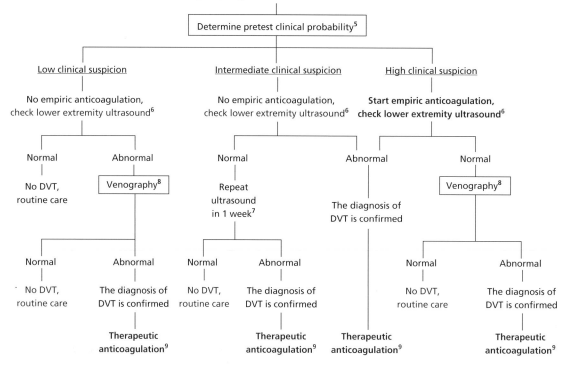

Suspect the diagnosis of deep vein thrombosis (DVT)[1]

- Take a detailed history and perform a physical examination[2]
- Be aware of pre-existing risk factors for DVT[3]
- Check CBC, T&S, coagulation studies[4]

Determine pretest clinical probability[5]

| Low clinical suspicion | Intermediate clinical suspicion | High clinical suspicion |

Low clinical suspicion — No empiric anticoagulation, check lower extremity ultrasound[6]

- Normal → No DVT, routine care
- Abnormal → Venography[8]
  - Normal → No DVT, routine care
  - Abnormal → The diagnosis of DVT is confirmed → Therapeutic anticoagulation[9]

Intermediate clinical suspicion — No empiric anticoagulation, check lower extremity ultrasound[6]

- Normal → Repeat ultrasound in 1 week[7]
  - Normal → No DVT, routine care
  - Abnormal → The diagnosis of DVT is confirmed → Therapeutic anticoagulation[9]
- Abnormal → The diagnosis of DVT is confirmed → Therapeutic anticoagulation[9]

High clinical suspicion — **Start empiric anticoagulation, check lower extremity ultrasound[6]**

- Normal → Venography[8]
  - Normal → No DVT, routine care
  - Abnormal → The diagnosis of DVT is confirmed → Therapeutic anticoagulation[9]

1. Venous thromboembolic events (VTE) – which includes both deep vein thrombosis (DVT) and pulmonary embolism (PE) – complicate 0.5–3.0 per 1000 pregnancies. VTE is the leading cause of maternal mortality in the Western world, accounting for 20–25% of pregnancy-related maternal deaths.

2. Symptoms suggestive of DVT include pain, swelling, and/or redness in the calf or thigh. Physical findings include objective evidence of calf swelling, localized redness, and calf tenderness with or without a palpable thrombotic "cord." Homan's sign refers to pain in the calf in response to active dorsiflexion of the foot. Pain in the calf is regarded as a "positive" Homan's sign and is taken to be suggestive of acute DVT. However, a "positive" Homan's sign is only around 30–40% sensitive, and a "negative" Homan's sign does not exclude the diagnosis.

3. Risk factors for VTE include inherited thrombophilia (such as factor V Leiden mutation, prothrombin gene mutation, protein/S/protein C/antithrombin deficiency), acquired thrombophilia (antiphospholipid antibody syndrome), advanced maternal age, increasing parity, obesity, prolonged immobility (bedrest), trauma (including surgery

Obstetric Clinical Algorithms: Management and Evidence. By © E.R. Norwitz, M. Belfort, G.R. Saade and H. Miller.
Published 2010 Blackwell Publishing.

such as cesarean delivery), and pregnancy. VTE is fivefold more common in pregnancy than in nonpregnant women, and is 3- to 5-fold more common in the puerperium and 3- to 16-fold more common after cesarean delivery.

4. Laboratory tests (including circulating D-dimer levels) are generally unhelpful in confirming the diagnosis of DVT, but baseline coagulation studies should be sent if the patient requires anticoagulation.

5. If the clinical suspicion of DVT is high, consider starting anticoagulation immediately to avoid DVT propagation and possible PE.

6. The diagnosis of DVT is usually confirmed noninvasively by venous ultrasonography, either B-mode or Doppler duplex, also known as lower extremity noninvasive (LENI) testing. Proximal lower extremity (thigh) DVT is evident in 25% of symptomatic patients, and is more commonly associated with PE. Distal lower extremity (calf) DVT is evident in 15% of symptomatic patients, but is rarely associated with PE. Venous ultrasonography is reliable at detecting proximal lower extremity DVT with a sensitivity of 95%, specificity of 96%, positive predictive value of 97%, and negative predictive value of 98%, but is less effective at diagnosing distal lower extremity DVT (sensitivity of 73%).

7. Venous ultrasonography is good at excluding proximal lower extremity DVT, but does not effectively exclude distal lower extremity DVT. As such, the minimal requirement in a symptomatic patient with a negative lower extremity venous ultrasound examination is to repeat the test in 1 week. By that time, 25% of symptomatic distal lower extremity thrombi will have extended into the proximal system.

8. If venous ultrasonography is negative, future management depends in large part on the clinical suspicion for DVT. If the clinical setting is highly suspicious, consider venography. Venography is the gold standard for the diagnosis of DVT, but is an invasive procedure. The contrast material can cause a chemical phlebitis. It can be performed in pregnancy so long as certain precautions are followed: adequate maternal hydration to facilitate renal clearance of the dye, and efforts to minimize pelvic irradiation (estimated amount of radiation exposure to the fetus is only 0.0005 Gy). *Consider venography if the clinical suspicion of DVT is low but venous ultrasonography is abnormal or if the clinical suspicion of DVT is high and ultrasonography is normal.*

9. Deep vein thrombosis in pregnancy should be treated to prevent propagation of the thrombus and PE. If untreated, 15–25% of patients with DVT will have a PE with a 15% mortality rate as compared with 4–5% of treated patients with a mortality rate of <1%. Therapeutic unfractionated heparin (UFH) is the treatment of choice for DVT in pregnancy. Treatment should be initiated with a loading dose of 100 U/kg (or minimum of 5000 U) followed by an initial infusion of 15–25 U/kg/h (or minimum of 1000 U/h). Serum PTT should be checked every 4 hours, and the infusion adjusted to maintain PTT at 1.5–2.5 × control. Once a steady state has been achieved, PTT levels should be measured daily. After 5–10 days, iv heparin can be changed to sc injection (not im injection because of the risk of hematoma) as follows: begin with 10,000 U sc tid and titrate dosage upward depending on the results of the PTT measured every 2–3 hours; aim for PTT 2.0–2.5 × control. Complications of UFH include hemorrhage, thrombocytopenia, osteopenia, and vertebral fracture. Heparins do not cross the placenta and, as such, are not teratogenic.

Although not well tested in pregnancy, existing data suggest that low molecular weight heparin (LMWH) may be as effective as UFH in the treatment of acute DVT in pregnancy. Examples of LMWH include enoxaparin (Lovenox) 1 mg/kg sc q12h and dalteparin (Fragmin) 150–200 U/kg sc q12h. LMWH does not significantly alter PTT, but serum anti-factor Xa activity can be measured. Therapeutic anticoagulation is achieved with a circulating anti-Xa activity of 0.6–1.0 U/mL. Similar to UFH, LMWH can be switched from IV to subcutaneous injection after 5–7 days as follows: enoxaparin (Lovenox) 1 mg/kg q 8–12 h or dalteparin (Fragmin) 200 U/kg q 8–12 h. LMWH has fewer side-effects than UFH. Alternative therapies (fibrinolytic agents, surgical intervention) are associated with a high incidence of complications in pregnancy and, as such, are best avoided.

Treatment for acute DVT should be continued throughout pregnancy and for at least 3–6 months postpartum. Oral coumadin (warfarin) is contraindicated in pregnancy (because it is teratogenic), but can be used postpartum. Whether all such women need antepartum anticoagulation in a subsequent pregnancy is unclear. Women with unexplained thrombosis and a confirmed thrombophilia may require prolonged anticoagulation.

10 Gestational Diabetes Mellitus[1,2]

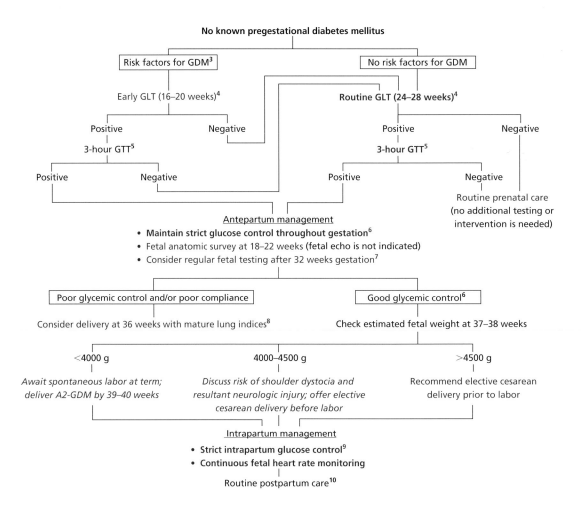

No known pregestational diabetes mellitus

Risk factors for GDM[3]

No risk factors for GDM

Early GLT (16–20 weeks)[4]

Routine GLT (24–28 weeks)[4]

Positive — 3-hour GTT[5]

Negative

Positive — 3-hour GTT[5]

Negative

Positive

Negative

Positive

Negative

Routine prenatal care
(no additional testing or
intervention is needed)

Antepartum management
- **Maintain strict glucose control throughout gestation[6]**
- Fetal anatomic survey at 18–22 weeks (fetal echo is not indicated)
- Consider regular fetal testing after 32 weeks gestation[7]

Poor glycemic control and/or poor compliance

Good glycemic control[6]

Consider delivery at 36 weeks with mature lung indices[8]

Check estimated fetal weight at 37–38 weeks

<4000 g

4000–4500 g

>4500 g

*Await spontaneous labor at term;
deliver A2-GDM by 39–40 weeks*

*Discuss risk of shoulder dystocia and
resultant neurologic injury; offer elective
cesarean delivery before labor*

*Recommend elective cesarean
delivery prior to labor*

Intrapartum management
- **Strict intrapartum glucose control[9]**
- **Continuous fetal heart rate monitoring**

Routine postpartum care[10]

Obstetric Clinical Algorithms: Management and Evidence. By © E.R. Norwitz, M. Belfort, G.R. Saade and H. Miller.
Published 2010 Blackwell Publishing.

1. Gestational diabetes (GDM) refers to glucose intolerance first detected during pregnancy. As such, it is likely that some patients diagnosed with GDM actually have unrecognized type II pregestational diabetes.

2. Pregnancy is a diabetogenic state with evidence of insulin resistance, maternal hyperinsulinism, and reduced peripheral uptake of glucose. This is due to high circulating levels of placental counter-regulatory (anti-insulin) hormones, including placental growth hormone and human chorionic somatomammotropins (previously known as human placental lactogens). These mechanisms ensure a continuous supply of glucose for the fetus. In some women, these changes unmask an underlying predisposition to insulin resistance leading to GDM. Depending on the population, 3–5% of pregnancies are complicated by GDM.

3. Risk factors for GDM include: a prior history of GDM, a family history (first-degree relative) of diabetes, a prior macrosomic or large-for-gestational age (LGA) infant, a prior unexplained late intrauterine fetal demise (IUFD), sustained glycosuria, hypertension or obesity. Such patients should have early testing for GDM at 16–20 weeks. If the early testing is negative, this should be repeated at 24–28 weeks.

4. Glucose load test (GLT) – also known as a glucose challenge test (GCT) – is a nonfasting test, but the woman should not eat after her 50 g glucose load until a venous blood sample is drawn 1 hour later. A value of ≥140 mg/dL (or less commonly ≥130 mg/dL) is considered positive and should be followed with a 3-hour glucose tolerance test (GTT); <2% of women with a GLT <140 mg/dL will have a positive GTT.

5. A definitive diagnosis of GDM requires a 3-hour GTT. There is no GLT cut-off that is diagnostic of GDM. Three days of carbohydrate loading is followed by a 100 g glucose load administered after an overnight fast. Venous plasma glucose is measured fasting and at 1 hour, 2 hours, and 3 hours. GDM requires two or more abnormal values defined as either ≥95, ≥180, ≥155, and ≥140 mg/dL, respectively (Carpenter & Coustan criteria) or ≥105, ≥190, ≥165, and ≥145 mg/dL, respectively (NDDG criteria). There is no place for HbA_{1c} to diagnose GDM.

6. The goal of antepartum management is to maintain strict glycemic control throughout gestation, defined as fasting blood glucose <95 mg/dL and 1-hour postprandial <140 mg/dL. A diabetic diet is recommended (defined as 36 kcal/kg or 15 kcal/lb of ideal bodyweight +100 kcal per trimester given as 40–50% carbohydrate, 20% protein, 30–40% fat) but, if diet alone does not maintain blood glucose at desirable levels, additional treatment may be needed. Insulin remains the "gold standard" although oral hypoglycemic agents (glyburide, glipizide) appear to be safe and effective and are being used more commonly as first-line agents. If fasting glucose levels are >95 mg/dL, treatment can be started right away because you "can't diet more than fasting."

7. Fetal testing is recommended for insulin-requiring GDM (class A2-GDM) after 32 weeks' gestation because of the risks of abnormal fetal growth (IUGR or macrosomia) and fetal demise. Testing should include daily fetal kick-charts, weekly nonstress testing, and serial ultrasound q 3–4 weeks for fetal growth.

8. If an elective delivery is planned prior to 39-0/7 weeks' gestation, ACOG mandates that fetal lung maturity is documented by amniocentesis prior to delivery using diabetes-specific cut-offs (such as L/S ratio ≥3.5, phosphatidylglycerol positive, TDx-FLM ≥55 mg surfactant per g of albumin).

9. During labor, patients are typically starved. Glucose should therefore be administered (5% dextrose iv at 75–100 mL/h) and blood glucose checked every 1–2 hours. Regular insulin is given as needed (either by subcutaneous injection or iv infusion) to maintain glucose at 100–120 mg/dL.

10. Delivery of the fetus and placenta removes the source of the anti-insulin hormones that causes GDM. As such, no further management is required in the immediate postpartum period. GDM likely unmasks an underlying predisposition for insulin resistance, and 40–60% of women with GDM will develop type 2 diabetes later in life. All women with GDM should therefore have a standard, nonpregnant 75 g GTT 6–8 weeks after delivery to exclude diabetes.

11 Gestational Hypertension[1]

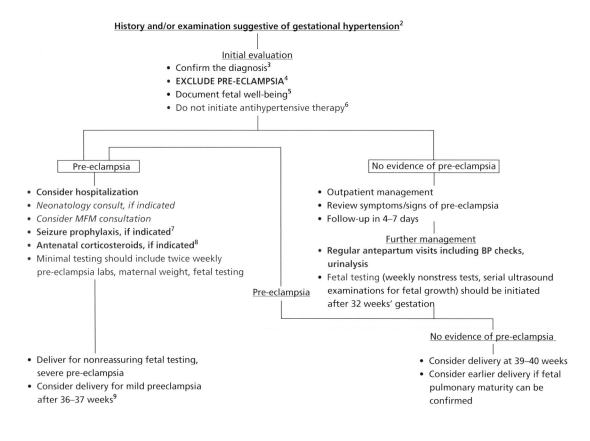

History and/or examination suggestive of gestational hypertension[2]

Initial evaluation
- Confirm the diagnosis[3]
- **EXCLUDE PRE-ECLAMPSIA**[4]
- **Document fetal well-being**[5]
- Do not initiate antihypertensive therapy[6]

Pre-eclampsia

- **Consider hospitalization**
- *Neonatology consult, if indicated*
- *Consider MFM consultation*
- **Seizure prophylaxis, if indicated**[7]
- **Antenatal corticosteroids, if indicated**[8]
- Minimal testing should include twice weekly pre-eclampsia labs, maternal weight, fetal testing

No evidence of pre-eclampsia

- Outpatient management
- Review symptoms/signs of pre-eclampsia
- Follow-up in 4–7 days

Further management
- **Regular antepartum visits including BP checks, urinalysis**
- Fetal testing (weekly nonstress tests, serial ultrasound examinations for fetal growth) should be initiated after 32 weeks' gestation

Pre-eclampsia

- Deliver for nonreassuring fetal testing, severe pre-eclampsia
- Consider delivery for mild preeclampsia after 36–37 weeks[9]

No evidence of pre-eclampsia

- Consider delivery at 39–40 weeks
- Consider earlier delivery if fetal pulmonary maturity can be confirmed

Obstetric Clinical Algorithms: Management and Evidence. By © E.R. Norwitz, M. Belfort, G.R. Saade and H. Miller.
Published 2010 Blackwell Publishing.

1. Also known as gestational nonproteinuric hypertension, pregnancy-induced hypertension (PIH).

2. Patients with gestational hypertension are typically asymptomatic. The diagnosis should be suspected in a patient who presents with a new-onset sustained elevation in BP≥140/90 without proteinuria in the third trimester.

3. Gestational hypertension refers to a sustained elevation in BP ≥ 140/90 mmHg without evidence of pre-eclampsia in a previously normotensive woman. It is a diagnosis which should only be made in the third trimester, and likely represents an exaggerated physiologic response of the maternal cardiovascular system to pregnancy.

4. Gestational hypertension is rarely associated with adverse maternal or fetal outcome. However, it is often difficult to distinguish prospectively from pre-eclampsia, which is a far more serious condition. As such, it is a diagnosis of exclusion and can only be made definitively in retrospect. The onus is therefore on the obstetric care provider to exclude pre-eclampsia. The following tests should be sent: urinalysis, 24-hour urine collection for protein quantitation and creatinine clearance, CBC, liver and renal function tests, and uric acid. It may be necessary to consider hospitalization to exclude pre-eclampsia. Even then, it may be a difficult distinction to make. It is known, for example, that 20% of women with eclampsia (and hence severe pre-eclampsia) do not have significant proteinuria prior to their seizure.

5. Such testing should include a nonstress test (looking for uteroplacental insufficiency), a BPP or amniotic fluid estimation, ultrasound for estimated fetal weight (EFW) or a combination of these modalities. Umbilical artery Doppler velocimetry is only useful in the setting of IUGR.

6. Treatment of mild hypertension has been shown not to improve pregnancy outcome. There are only three indications for antihypertensive therapy in pregnancy: (i) established or suspected underlying chronic hypertension; (ii) to achieve BP control to prevent cerebrovascular accident while effecting delivery; and/or (iii) expectant management of severe pre-eclampsia by BP criteria alone less than 32 weeks (Sibai protocol).

7. Intravenous magnesium sulfate is the drug of choice and should be given intrapartum and for at least 24 hours postpartum to prevent eclampsia. Antenatal corticosteroids are rarely indicated for gestational hypertension, because it is typically a diagnosis of the late third trimester and antenatal corticosteroids have no proven benefit after 34 weeks. Delivery is the only effective treatment for pre-eclampsia. It is recommended in women with mild pre-eclampsia once a favorable gestational age has been reached and in all women with severe pre-eclampsia regardless of gestational age (with the exception of severe pre-eclampsia due to proteinuria alone, IUGR remote from term with good fetal testing, or possibly severe pre-eclampsia by BP criteria alone <32 weeks (Sibai protocol)). There is no proven benefit to routine delivery by cesarean. However, the probability of vaginal delivery in a patient with pre-eclampsia remote from term with an unfavorable cervix is only 15–20%. Pre-eclampsia and its complications always resolve following delivery (with the exception of stroke). Diuresis (>4 L/day) is the most accurate clinical indicator of resolution. Fetal prognosis is dependent largely on gestational age at delivery.

12 Pre-eclampsia

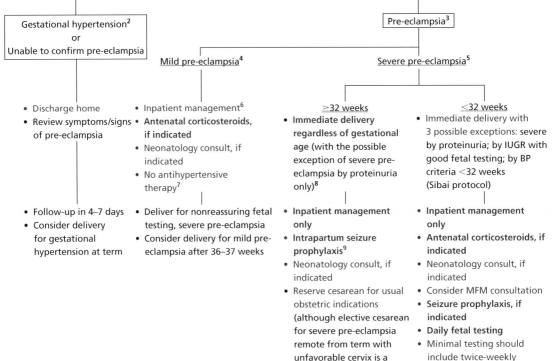

History and/or examination suggestive of pre-eclampsia[1]

Further evaluation
- Check serial sitting BP, pre-eclampsia labs, urinalysis
- Assess fetal well-being
- Consider evaluation on L&D and/or admission to observation for 24–48 hours

Gestational hypertension[2]
or
Unable to confirm pre-eclampsia

Pre-eclampsia[3]

Mild pre-eclampsia[4]

Severe pre-eclampsia[5]

- Discharge home
- Review symptoms/signs of pre-eclampsia

- Follow-up in 4–7 days
- Consider delivery for gestational hypertension at term

- Inpatient management[6]
- **Antenatal corticosteroids, if indicated**
- Neonatology consult, if indicated
- No antihypertensive therapy[7]

- Deliver for nonreassuring fetal testing, severe pre-eclampsia
- Consider delivery for mild pre-eclampsia after 36–37 weeks

≥32 weeks
- **Immediate delivery regardless of gestational age (with the possible exception of severe pre-eclampsia by proteinuria only)[8]**

- **Inpatient management only**
- **Intrapartum seizure prophylaxis[9]**
- Neonatology consult, if indicated
- Reserve cesarean for usual obstetric indications (although elective cesarean for severe pre-eclampsia remote from term with unfavorable cervix is a reasonable option)

<32 weeks
- Immediate delivery with 3 possible exceptions: severe by proteinuria; by IUGR with good fetal testing; by BP criteria <32 weeks (Sibai protocol)

- **Inpatient management only**
- **Antenatal corticosteroids, if indicated**
- Neonatology consult, if indicated
- Consider MFM consultation
- **Seizure prophylaxis, if indicated**
- **Daily fetal testing**
- Minimal testing should include twice-weekly pre-eclampsia labs, maternal weight
- Consider delivery ≥34 weeks

Obstetric Clinical Algorithms: Management and Evidence. By © E.R. Norwitz, M. Belfort, G.R. Saade and H. Miller.
Published 2010 Blackwell Publishing.

1. Most patients are asymptomatic. Symptoms may include headache, visual aberrations, and right upper quadrant or epigastric pain. Signs may include elevated BP, excessive weight gain, nondependent edema, brisk deep tendon reflexes or excessive clonus, and right upper quadrant or epigastric tenderness.

2. Also known as nonproteinuric hypertension or pregnancy-induced hypertension (PIH). Refers to a persistent elevation of BP $\geq$ 140/90 mmHg in the third trimester without evidence of pre-eclampsia in a previously normotensive woman. It is a diagnosis of exclusion, and likely represents an exaggerated physiologic response of the maternal cardiovascular system to pregnancy. It is rarely associated with adverse events, but can be difficult to distinguish prospectively from pre-eclampsia.

3. Also known as gestational proteinuric hypertension or pre-eclamptic toxemia (PET). Pre-eclampsia is a multisystem disorder specific to pregnancy and the puerperium. More precisely, it is a disease of the placenta since it occurs in pregnancies where there is trophoblast but no fetal tissue (complete molar pregnancies). Pre-eclampsia is a <u>clinical</u> diagnosis with three elements: (i) new-onset hypertension defined as a sustained BP $\geq$ 140/90 mmHg in a previously normotensive woman (a prior definition included an elevation in systolic BP $\geq$ 30 or diastolic BP $\geq$ 15 mmHg over first-trimester BP, but these criteria have now been dropped); (ii) new-onset significant proteinuria defined as >300 mg/24 h or $\geq$1+ on a clean-catch urine in the absence of urinary tract infection; and (iii) new-onset nondependent edema (swelling of face and hands). Nondependent edema is not a prerequisite for the diagnosis. A definitive diagnosis of pre-eclampsia should only be made after 20 weeks' gestation. Evidence of gestational proteinuric hypertension prior to 20 weeks should raise the possibility of an underlying molar pregnancy, drug withdrawal or (rarely) chromosomal abnormality in the fetus.

4. Refers to all women who fulfil the criteria for pre-eclampsia without any criteria for severe pre-eclampsia.

5. Refers to all women who fulfil the criteria for pre-eclampsia with one or more of the following:
- symptoms (headache, visual aberrations, right upper quadrant pain)
- signs (BP $\geq$ 160/110 mmHg on two occasions at least 6 h apart, seizures or coma (eclampsia), pulmonary edema, ARDS, cardiac failure, stroke, cortical blindness, oliguria, IUGR, liver hematoma or rupture)
- laboratory tests (thrombocytopenia, serum transaminase levels $\geq$2 $\times$ normal, HELLP syndrome, proteinuria >5 g/day, renal failure, DIC)

6. Outpatient management of mild pre-eclampsia may be an option for a limited number of patients if all of the following criteria can be met: patient lives close to a hospital, has someone with her at all times, can be on strict bedrest at home, daily visiting nurse for BP checks, daily kickcharts, twice-weekly outpatient visits for pre-eclampsia labs and fetal testing, both patient and physician are comfortable with the plan and understand the risks, and patient will report symptoms of severe pre-eclampsia immediately.

7. There are only three indications for antihypertensive therapy in the setting of pre-eclampsia: (i) underlying chronic hypertension; (ii) to achieve BP control to prevent cerebrovascular accident while effecting delivery; and/or (iii) expectant management of severe pre-eclampsia by BP criteria alone (Sibai protocol). BP control is important to prevent cerebrovascular accident (usually associated with BP $\geq$ 170/120 mmHg), but does not affect the natural course of pre-eclampsia.

8. Delivery is the only effective treatment, It is recommended in women with mild pre-eclampsia once a favorable gestational age has been reached and in all women with severe pre-eclampsia regardless of gestational age (with the exception of severe pre-eclampsia due to proteinuria alone or IUGR remote from term with good fetal testing). There has also been a recent trend towards expectant management of severe pre-eclampsia by BP criteria alone <32 weeks (Sibai protocol). There is no proven benefit to routine delivery by cesarean. However, the probability of vaginal delivery in a patient with pre-eclampsia remote from term with an unfavorable cervix is only 15–20%. Pre-eclampsia and its complications always resolve following delivery (with the exception of stroke). Diuresis (>4 L/day) is the most accurate clinical indicator of resolution. Fetal prognosis is dependent largely on gestational age at delivery.

9. Intravenous magnesium sulfate is the drug of choice and should be given intrapartum and for at least 24 hours postpartum to prevent eclampsia.

13 Pregestational Diabetes Mellitus

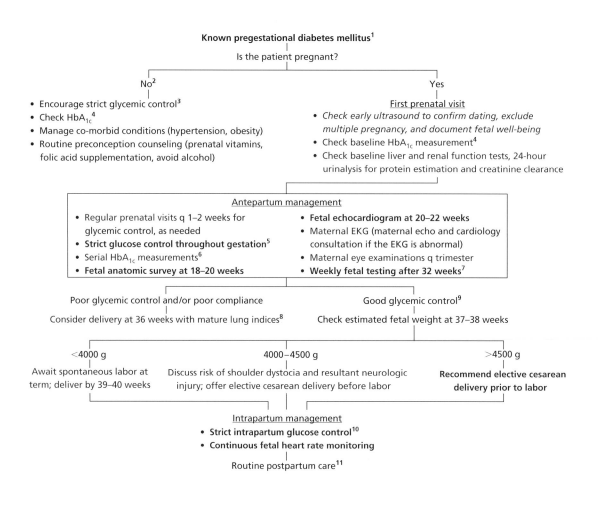

Known pregestational diabetes mellitus[1]

Is the patient pregnant?

No[2]

- Encourage strict glycemic control[3]
- Check HbA$_{1c}$[4]
- Manage co-morbid conditions (hypertension, obesity)
- Routine preconception counseling (prenatal vitamins, folic acid supplementation, avoid alcohol)

Yes

First prenatal visit

- *Check early ultrasound to confirm dating, exclude multiple pregnancy, and document fetal well-being*
- Check baseline HbA$_{1c}$ measurement[4]
- Check baseline liver and renal function tests, 24-hour urinalysis for protein estimation and creatinine clearance

Antepartum management

- Regular prenatal visits q 1–2 weeks for glycemic control, as needed
- **Strict glucose control throughout gestation[5]**
- Serial HbA$_{1c}$ measurements[6]
- **Fetal anatomic survey at 18–20 weeks**
- **Fetal echocardiogram at 20–22 weeks**
- Maternal EKG (maternal echo and cardiology consultation if the EKG is abnormal)
- Maternal eye examinations q trimester
- **Weekly fetal testing after 32 weeks[7]**

Poor glycemic control and/or poor compliance

Consider delivery at 36 weeks with mature lung indices[8]

Good glycemic control[9]

Check estimated fetal weight at 37–38 weeks

<4000 g

Await spontaneous labor at term; deliver by 39–40 weeks

4000–4500 g

Discuss risk of shoulder dystocia and resultant neurologic injury; offer elective cesarean delivery before labor

>4500 g

Recommend elective cesarean delivery prior to labor

Intrapartum management

- **Strict intrapartum glucose control[10]**
- **Continuous fetal heart rate monitoring**

Routine postpartum care[11]

Obstetric Clinical Algorithms: Management and Evidence. By © E.R. Norwitz, M. Belfort, G.R. Saade and H. Miller.
Published 2010 Blackwell Publishing.

1. Pregestational diabetes results from either an absolute deficiency of insulin (type 1, insulin-dependent diabetes mellitus) or increased peripheral resistance to insulin (type 2, noninsulin-dependent diabetes mellitus (NIDDM)). It complicates <1% of women of childbearing age. The age of onset and duration of diabetes (White classification) do not correlate with pregnancy outcome. Poor prognostic features include a history of diabetic ketoacidosis (DKA), poor compliance, poorly controlled hypertension, pyelonephritis, and vasculopathy.

2. Pregestational diabetes is associated with significant maternal and perinatal mortality and morbidity. Diabetic women should ideally be seen prior to conception. Pregnancy complications such as fetal congenital anomalies (diabetic embryopathy) and spontaneous abortion correlate directly with the degree of diabetic control around the time of conception.

3. Strict glycemic control is defined as fasting blood glucose <95 mg/dL and 1-hour postprandial <140 mg/dL (or 2-hour postprandial <120 mg/dL).

4. Approximately 5% of maternal hemoglobin is glycosylated (bound to glucose). This fraction is known as hemoglobin A1 (HbA1). HbA_{1c} refers to the 80–85% of HbA1 that is irreversibly glycosylated and, as such, is a more reliable and reproducible measurement. Since red blood cells have a lifespan of 120 days, HbA_{1c} measurements reflect the degree of glycemic control over the prior 3–4 months. A normal HbA_{1c} varies from laboratory to laboratory, but is typically <5.9%.

5. The goal of antepartum management is to maintain strict glycemic control throughout gestation, defined as fasting blood glucose <95 mg/dL and 1-hour postprandial <140 mg/dL (or 2-hour postprandial <120 mg/dL). A diabetic diet is recommended (defined as 36 kcal/kg or 15 kcal/lb of ideal bodyweight +100 kcal per trimester given as 40–50% carbohydrate, 20% protein, 30–40% fat), but if diet alone does not maintain blood glucose at desirable levels, additional treatment may be needed. Insulin remains the "gold standard" although oral hypoglycemic agents (glyburide, glipizide) appear to be safe and effective and are being used more commonly as first-line agents. If fasting glucose levels are >95 mg/dL, treatment can be started right away *because you can't diet more than fasting."* Intense antepartum management and strict glycemic control can reduce perinatal mortality from 20% to 3–5%.

6. HbA_{1c} measurements should be checked prior to conception, at first prenatal visit, and every 4–6 weeks throughout pregnancy.

7. Fetal testing is recommended in all cases of pregestational diabetes after 32 weeks' gestation because of the risks of abnormal fetal growth (intrauterine growth restriction or macrosomia), abnormal amniotic fluid volume, and fetal demise. Testing should include daily fetal kickcharts, weekly nonstress testing (NST) with or without sonographic estimation of amniotic fluid volume, and serial ultrasound q 3–4 weeks for fetal growth.

8. If an elective delivery is planned prior to 39–0/7 weeks gestation, ACOG mandates that fetal lung maturity is documented by amniocentesis prior to delivery using diabetes-specific cut-offs (such as L/S ratio ≥ 3.5, phosphatidylglycerol positive, TDx-FLM $\geq$ 55 mg surfactant per g of albumin).

9. If metabolic control is good, spontaneous labor at term can be awaited. Because of the risk of unexplained fetal demise, women with pregestational diabetes should be delivered by 39–40 weeks.

10. During labor, patients are typically starved. Glucose should therefore be administered (5% dextrose iv at 75–100 mL/h) and blood glucose checked every 1–2 hours. Regular insulin is given as needed (either by subcutaneous injection or iv infusion) to maintain glucose at 100–120 mg/dL.

11. During the first 48 hours postpartum, women may have a "honeymoon period" during which their insulin requirement is decreased. Blood glucose levels of 150–200 mg/dL (8.2–11.0 mmol/L) can be tolerated during this period. Once a woman is able to eat, she can be placed back on her regular insulin regimen.

14 Pulmonary Edema

Pulmonary edema[1]

Confirm the diagnosis

- Identify risk factors for pulmonary edema[2]
- Take a detailed history and perform a physical examination[3]
- √ chest x-ray
- Consider alternative diagnoses[4]

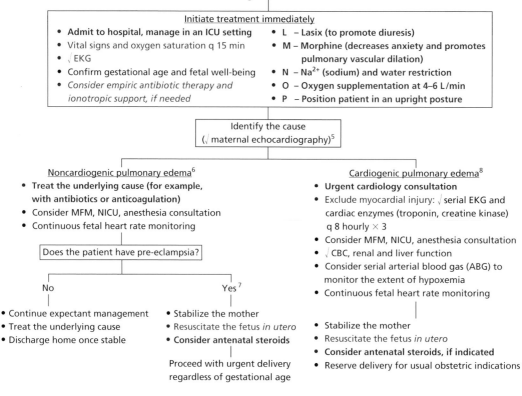

Initiate treatment immediately

- Admit to hospital, manage in an ICU setting
- Vital signs and oxygen saturation q 15 min
- √ EKG
- Confirm gestational age and fetal well-being
- *Consider empiric antibiotic therapy and ionotropic support, if needed*

- L – Lasix (to promote diuresis)
- M – Morphine (decreases anxiety and promotes pulmonary vascular dilation)
- N – Na^{2+} (sodium) and water restriction
- O – Oxygen supplementation at 4–6 L/min
- P – Position patient in an upright posture

Identify the cause
(√ maternal echocardiography)[5]

Noncardiogenic pulmonary edema[6]
- **Treat the underlying cause (for example, with antibiotics or anticoagulation)**
- Consider MFM, NICU, anesthesia consultation
- Continuous fetal heart rate monitoring

Does the patient have pre-eclampsia?

No | Yes[7]

No:
- Continue expectant management
- Treat the underlying cause
- Discharge home once stable

Yes:
- Stabilize the mother
- *Resuscitate the fetus in utero*
- **Consider antenatal steroids**

Proceed with urgent delivery regardless of gestational age

Cardiogenic pulmonary edema[8]
- **Urgent cardiology consultation**
- Exclude myocardial injury: √ serial EKG and cardiac enzymes (troponin, creatine kinase) q 8 hourly × 3
- Consider MFM, NICU, anesthesia consultation
- √ CBC, renal and liver function
- Consider serial arterial blood gas (ABG) to monitor the extent of hypoxemia
- Continuous fetal heart rate monitoring

- Stabilize the mother
- *Resuscitate the fetus in utero*
- **Consider antenatal steroids, if indicated**
- Reserve delivery for usual obstetric indications

Obstetric Clinical Algorithms: Management and Evidence. By © E.R. Norwitz, M. Belfort, G.R. Saade and H. Miller.
Published 2010 Blackwell Publishing.

1. Pulmonary edema refers to an abnormal and excessive accumulation of fluid in the alveolar and interstitial spaces of the lungs.

2. Risk factors for pulmonary edema include pre-eclampsia, infection, iatrogenic fluid overload, and tocolytic therapy (such as β-agonist medications).

3. Accumulation of fluid in the alveolar space leads to decreased diffusing capacity, hypoxemia, and shortness of breath (dyspnea). Patients present with worsening dyspnea and orthopnea (inability to lie flat) which may be acute or slowly progressive in onset. Other symptoms may include cough, chest pain, palpitations, fatigue, and low-grade fever. Physical examination may reveal tachycardia, elevated blood pressure, and peripheral edema. Cardiac evaluation may uncover an irregular heart beat, elevated jugular venous pressure (which reflects an elevated right-sided filling pressure), and the presence of a S3 or S4 heart sound or both ("summation gallop") as well as a new or changed heart murmur. Chest examination usually reveals crackles indicative of interstitial pulmonary edema and some patients may have wheezing ("cardiac asthma"). The diagnosis is typically confirmed on chest radiograph. Radiographic findings can range from mild pulmonary vascular redistribution to extensive bilateral interstitial marking and pleural effusions. The presence of bilateral perihilar alveolar edema may give the typical "butterfly" appearance. The presence of cardiomegaly suggests a cardiac cause.

4. Consider alternative diagnoses, including pulmonary embolism (see Chapter 15), severe asthma exacerbation, and pneumonia.

5. All pregnant women with pulmonary edema should have a maternal echocardiogram (ideally a transesophageal echo) to exclude underlying cardiac disease.

6. *Noncardiogenic pulmonary edema* is defined as radiographic evidence of fluid and protein accumulation in the alveolar space of the lungs without evidence of a cardiogenic cause (i.e. a normal maternal echo and pulmonary capillary wedge pressure <18 mmHg). The major causes of noncardiogenic pulmonary edema include: the acute respiratory distress syndrome (ARDS) and, less often, high-altitude pulmonary edema, neurogenic pulmonary edema, pulmonary embolism, salicylate toxicity, opiate overdose, pre-eclampsia, amniotic fluid embolism, and reperfusion pulmonary edema. ARDS can develop as a result of a number of insults, including sepsis, acute pulmonary infection, nonthoracic trauma, inhaled toxins, disseminated intravascular coagulation, shock lung, free-base cocaine smoking, postcoronary artery bypass grafting, inhalation of high oxygen concentrations, and acute radiation pneumonia. Hypoalbuminemia alone is not a cause of noncardiogenic pulmonary edema. The primary pathophysiologic mechanism of noncardiogenic pulmonary edema is an increase in capillary permeability. Treatment is primarily supportive care.

7. If the patient has pre-eclampsia (gestational proteinuric hypertension), the presence of pulmonary edema puts her in the "severe pre-eclampsia" category (see Chapter 12) and is a contraindication to continued expectant management. Immediate delivery should be recommended regardless of gestational age. Whether delivery can be delayed for 24–48 hours to complete a course of antenatal corticosteroids in women remote from term (<34 weeks) should be individualized.

8. *Cardiogenic pulmonary edema* is characterized by increased transudation of protein-poor fluid into the pulmonary interstitium and alveolar space. Fluid transudation results from a rise in pulmonary capillary pressure (as measured by pulmonary capillary wedge pressure ≥18 mmHg) due to an increase in pulmonary venous and left atrial pressures. This typically occurs in the absence of a change in vascular integrity or permeability. The major causes of cardiogenic pulmonary edema include: myocardial injury or infarction, valvular heart disease, cardiomyopathy, cardiac arrhythmia, poorly controlled systemic hypertension, and, less often, severe anemia, thyroid disease, toxins such as cocaine and alcohol, fever, intercurrent infection (such as pneumonia), and uncontrolled diabetes.

15 Pulmonary Embolism[1]

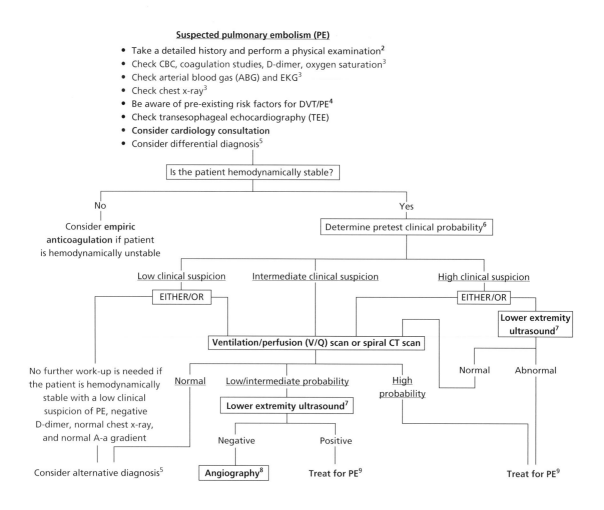

Suspected pulmonary embolism (PE)
- Take a detailed history and perform a physical examination[2]
- Check CBC, coagulation studies, D-dimer, oxygen saturation[3]
- Check arterial blood gas (ABG) and EKG[3]
- Check chest x-ray[3]
- Be aware of pre-existing risk factors for DVT/PE[4]
- Check transesophageal echocardiography (TEE)
- **Consider cardiology consultation**
- Consider differential diagnosis[5]

Is the patient hemodynamically stable?

No

Consider **empiric anticoagulation** if patient is hemodynamically unstable

Yes

Determine pretest clinical probability[6]

Low clinical suspicion

EITHER/OR

Intermediate clinical suspicion

High clinical suspicion

EITHER/OR

Lower extremity ultrasound[7]

Ventilation/perfusion (V/Q) scan or spiral CT scan

No further work-up is needed if the patient is hemodynamically stable with a low clinical suspicion of PE, negative D-dimer, normal chest x-ray, and normal A-a gradient

Normal

Low/intermediate probability

High probability

Normal

Abnormal

Lower extremity ultrasound[7]

Consider alternative diagnosis[5]

Negative

Positive

Angiography[8]

Treat for PE[9]

Treat for PE[9]

Obstetric Clinical Algorithms: Management and Evidence. By © E.R. Norwitz, M. Belfort, G.R. Saade and H. Miller. Published 2010 Blackwell Publishing.

1. Venous thromboembolic events (VTE) – which includes both deep vein thrombosis (DVT) and pulmonary embolism (PE) – complicate 0.5–3.0 per 1000 pregnancies. VTE is the leading cause of maternal mortality in the Western world, accounting for 20–25% of pregnancy-related maternal deaths.

2. Symptoms of PE include acute-onset shortness of breath (dyspnea), pleuritic chest pain, cough, and/or hemoptysis. Physical signs suggestive of PE may include low-grade fever, tachypnea, tachycardia, diminished oxygen saturation, diminished breath sounds, audible crackles and/or evidence of pleural effusion on pulmonary examination. The single most sensitive sign of pulmonary embolism is unexplained tachycardia, although it is nonspecific.

3. Laboratory tests may reveal acidosis and an elevated A-a gradient on ABG analysis and evidence of right heart strain on EKG (S1Q3T3 pattern with or without right axis deviation, T wave inversion) on EKG. CXR may be normal or show evidence of multiple peripheral wedge-shaped areas of consolidation, pulmonary edema, and/or pleural effusion. Note that ABG, EKG, and CXR lack sufficient specificity to make the diagnosis. However, if ABG reveals an arterial pO_2 >80 mmHg, the diagnosis of PE is highly unlikely. Similarly, although D-dimer levels are not generally helpful in making the diagnosis of PE, a clinically significant VTE is highly unlikely if the D-dimer is normal.

4. Risk factors for VTE are summarized in Chapter 9.

5. The differential diagnosis of PE includes pneumonia, pneumothorax, congestive cardiac failure, pericarditis, pulmonary edema, and rib fracture.

6. If the clinical suspicion for acute PE is high, consider starting therapeutic anticoagulation immediately to avoid clot propagation and possible repeat PE.

7. The diagnosis of DVT is usually confirmed noninvasively by venous ultrasonography, also known as lower extremity noninvasive (LENI) testing. If there is a high clinical suspicion for PE and a confirmed DVT on LENI, it is reasonable to make a diagnosis of PE without further testing and treat accordingly. Similarly, if there is an intermediate clinical suspicion for PE and a low/intermediate probability of PE on ventilation/perfusion (V/Q) scan, it is also reasonable to make a diagnosis of PE without further testing and treat accordingly.

8. Pulmonary angiography is the "gold standard" for the diagnosis of acute PE, but is an invasive procedure. Angiography can be performed in pregnancy so long as certain precautions are followed: adequate maternal hydration to facilitate renal clearance of the dye, and efforts to minimize pelvic irradiation. Consider angiography only if the clinical suspicion of PE is low but V/Q scan is abnormal (that is, there is a ventilation/perfusion mismatch) or if the clinical suspicion of PE is high and the V/Q scan is normal. CT scan (especially spiral CT scan) is being used increasingly for the diagnosis of PE.

9. Therapeutic <u>unfractionated heparin</u> (UFH) is the treatment of choice for acute PE in pregnancy. Treatment should be initiated with a loading dose of 150 U/kg (or minimum of 5000 U) followed by an initial infusion of 15-25 U/kg/h (or minimum of 1000 U/h). Serum PTT should be checked every 4 hours, and the infusion adjusted to maintain PTT at 1.5–2.5 × control. Once a steady state has been achieved, PTT levels should be measured daily. After 5–10 days, iv heparin can be changed to subcutaneous injection (not intramuscular injection because of the risk of hematoma) as follows: begin with 10,000 U sc tid and titrate dosage upward depending on the results of the PTT measured every 2–3 hours; aim for PTT 2.0–2.5 × control. Complications of UFH include hemorrhage, thrombocytopenia, osteopenia, and vertebral fracture. Heparins do not cross the placenta and, as such, are not teratogenic.

Existing data suggest that <u>low molecular weight heparin</u> (LMWH) may be as effective as UFH in the treatment of PE in pregnancy. Examples of LMWH include enoxaparin (Lovenox) 1 mg/kg sc q12h and dalteparin (Fragmin) 150–200 U/kg sc q12h. LMWH does not significantly alter PTT, but serum anti-factor Xa activity can be measured. Therapeutic anticoagulation is achieved with a circulating anti-Xa activity of 0.6–1.0 U/mL. Similar to UFH, LMWH can be switched from iv to sc injection after 5–7 days. LMWH has fewer side-effects than UFH. Alternative therapies (fibrinolytic agents, surgical intervention) are associated with a high incidence of complications in pregnancy and, as such, are best avoided.

Treatment should be continued throughout pregnancy and for at least 3–6 months postpartum. Oral coumadin (warfarin) is contraindicated in pregnancy (because it is teratogenic), but can be used postpartum. Whether all such women need antepartum anticoagulation in a subsequent pregnancy is unclear.

16 Renal Disease

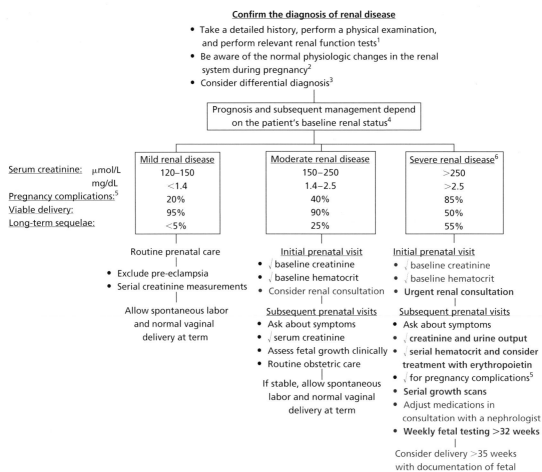

Confirm the diagnosis of renal disease

- Take a detailed history, perform a physical examination, and perform relevant renal function tests[1]
- Be aware of the normal physiologic changes in the renal system during pregnancy[2]
- Consider differential diagnosis[3]

Prognosis and subsequent management depend on the patient's baseline renal status[4]

Serum creatinine: µmol/L
                   mg/dL
Pregnancy complications:[5]
Viable delivery:
Long-term sequelae:

	Mild renal disease	Moderate renal disease	Severe renal disease[6]
µmol/L	120–150	150–250	>250
mg/dL	<1.4	1.4–2.5	>2.5
Pregnancy complications	20%	40%	85%
Viable delivery	95%	90%	50%
Long-term sequelae	<5%	25%	55%

Mild renal disease

Routine prenatal care

- Exclude pre-eclampsia
- Serial creatinine measurements

Allow spontaneous labor and normal vaginal delivery at term

Moderate renal disease

Initial prenatal visit
- √ baseline creatinine
- √ baseline hematocrit
- Consider renal consultation

Subsequent prenatal visits
- Ask about symptoms
- √ serum creatinine
- Assess fetal growth clinically
- Routine obstetric care

If stable, allow spontaneous labor and normal vaginal delivery at term

Severe renal disease

Initial prenatal visit
- √ baseline creatinine
- √ baseline hematocrit
- **Urgent renal consultation**

Subsequent prenatal visits
- Ask about symptoms
- √ **creatinine and urine output**
- √ **serial hematocrit and consider treatment with erythropoietin**
- √ **for pregnancy complications[5]**
- **Serial growth scans**
- Adjust medications in consultation with a nephrologist
- **Weekly fetal testing >32 weeks**

Consider delivery >35 weeks with documentation of fetal lung maturation

Obstetric Clinical Algorithms: Management and Evidence. By © E.R. Norwitz, M. Belfort, G.R. Saade and H. Miller.
Published 2010 Blackwell Publishing.

1. A number of renal disorders can complicate pregnancy. Asymptomatic bacteriuria (Chapter 21) and urinary tract infection/pyelonephritis (Chapter 22) are dealt with elsewhere in this book. Acute and chronic renal disease may be asymptomatic or may present with complaints of oliguria/polyuria, frequency, urgency, and pain or bleeding on urination. Renal function tests useful in diagnosing and following renal disease include serum and urine creatinine and urea (blood urea nitrogen (BUN)) measurements, BUN/creatinine ratio, fractional excretion of sodium (FeNa), and 24-hour urinary collections for protein estimation and creatinine clearance. In general, women with mild, well-controlled renal disease tolerate pregnancy well. Women with severe renal disease are at risk of symptomatic deterioration and end-stage renal insufficiency.

2. A number of changes occur in the genitourinary system during pregnancy. The glomerular filtration rate (GFR) increases by 50% early in pregnancy, leading to an increase in creatinine clearance and a 25% decrease in serum creatinine and urea concentrations. The increased GFR results in an increase in filtered sodium, and aldosterone levels increase 2–3-fold to reabsorb this sodium. The increased GFR also results in decreased resorption of glucose; as such, 15% of normal pregnant women exhibit glycosuria. Mild hydronephrosis and hydroureter are common sonographic findings due to both high levels of progesterone (which is a smooth muscle relaxant) and partial obstruction of the ureters by the gravid uterus at the level of the pelvic brim.

As regards the fetal genitourinary system, fetal urination starts early in pregnancy and fetal urine is a major component of amniotic fluid, especially after 16 weeks. Fetal renal function improves slowly as pregnancy progresses. Until delivery, the placenta performs much of the waste disposal responsibilities.

3. The differential diagnosis of intrinsic renal insufficiency includes dehydration, renal artery stenosis, pre-renal disorders (hypovolemic or septic shock, congestive cardiac failure), obstructive uropathy (renal stone, postoperative stricture or obstruction), and endocrine disorders such as syndrome of inappropriate ADH secretion (SIADH), diabetes insipidus, hyperaldosteronism, and Cushing syndrome.

4. Pregnancy outcome depends on baseline renal function (above) and on the presence and severity of hypertension. The degree of proteinuria does not correlate with pregnancy outcome.

5. Pregnancy-related complications of renal disease include infertility (due usually to chronic anovulation), spontaneous abortion, pre-eclampsia, intrauterine growth restriction (IUGR), stillbirth/intrauterine fetal demise (IUFD), and spontaneous preterm birth.

6. In women with end-stage renal disease, renal transplantation offers the best chance of a pregnancy success, especially if renal function is stable for 1–2 years after transplantation and there is no hypertension. Triple-agent immunosuppression (cyclosporine, azathioprine, and prednisone) should be continued during pregnancy.

17 Seizure Disorder

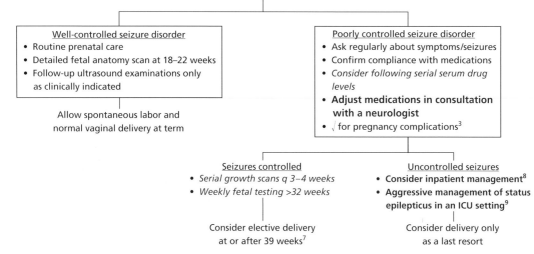

Confirm the diagnosis of seizure disorder[1]
- Take a detailed history and perform a physical examination
- Be aware of the effects of pregnancy on seizure disorder[2]
- Be aware of the effects of seizure disorders on pregnancy[3]
- Consider differential diagnosis[4]

Preconception counseling
- Review the risks of a seizure disorder and anticonvulsant medications with the couple[5]
- **Manage in consultation with a neurologist[6]**
- **Start folic acid supplementation[5]**

First prenatal visit
- Confirm gestational age and fetal well-being
- √ baseline liver and renal function tests
- Arrange regular prenatal and neurology follow-up

Well-controlled seizure disorder
- Routine prenatal care
- Detailed fetal anatomy scan at 18–22 weeks
- Follow-up ultrasound examinations only as clinically indicated

Allow spontaneous labor and normal vaginal delivery at term

Poorly controlled seizure disorder
- Ask regularly about symptoms/seizures
- Confirm compliance with medications
- *Consider following serial serum drug levels*
- **Adjust medications in consultation with a neurologist**
- √ for pregnancy complications[3]

Seizures controlled
- *Serial growth scans q 3–4 weeks*
- *Weekly fetal testing >32 weeks*

Consider elective delivery at or after 39 weeks[7]

Uncontrolled seizures
- **Consider inpatient management[8]**
- **Aggressive management of status epilepticus in an ICU setting[9]**

Consider delivery only as a last resort

Obstetric Clinical Algorithms: Management and Evidence. By © E.R. Norwitz, M. Belfort, G.R. Saade and H. Miller.
Published 2010 Blackwell Publishing.

1. Seizure disorders are the most frequently encountered major neurologic condition in pregnancy, affecting 0.3–0.6% of all gestations. Seizures can be classified into primary (idiopathic, epilepsy) or secondary (to trauma, infection, tumors, cerebrovascular disease, drug withdrawal, metabolic disorders or pre-eclampsia/eclampsia).

2. The effect of pregnancy on seizure disorders is variable. High estrogen levels lower the seizure threshold, while progesterone raises it. Seizure frequency is increased in 45% of pregnant women, reduced in 5%, and unchanged in 50%. If seizures are well controlled prior to pregnancy, there is little risk of deterioration. However, if poorly controlled, an increase in seizure frequency can be expected. Moreover, due to a number of factors (including delayed gastric emptying, increase in plasma volume, altered protein binding, and accelerated hepatic metabolism), the pharmacokinetics of anticonvulsant drugs change during pregnancy.

3. A number of obstetric complications are more common in women with epilepsy, including an increased risk of hyperemesis gravidarum, spontaneous abortion, spontaneous preterm delivery, pre-eclampsia/eclampsia, cesarean delivery, placental abruption, and perinatal mortality. However, the majority of women with seizure disorders will have an uneventful pregnancy.

4. The differential diagnosis of idiopathic seizures (epilepsy) includes drug withdrawal, intracranial lesions (including tumors and intracerebral hemorrhage), trauma, infection, metabolic disorders, and pseudo-seizures. All seizures in pregnancy should be regarded as pre-eclampsia/eclampsia until proven otherwise.

5. Women with epilepsy have a 2–3-fold increased incidence of fetal anomalies even off treatment. Moreover, anticonvulsant drugs are teratogenic (see Chapter 55). The incidence of fetal anomalies increases with the number of anticonvulsant drugs: 3–4% with one, 5–6% with two, 10% with three, and 25% with four. Monotherapy is thus recommended. *Valproic acid* is associated with neural tube defects (NTD) in 1% of cases. Risk is greatest from days 17–30 postconception (days 31–44 from LMP). Folic acid (4 mg daily) decreases the incidence of NTD tenfold to a baseline risk of 0.1%. 10–30% of women on *phenytoin* will have infants with one or more of the following features: craniofacial abnormalities (cleft lip, epicanthic folds, hypertelorism), cardiac anomalies, limb defects (hypoplasia of distal phalanges, nail hypoplasia), or IUGR. "Fetal hydantoin syndrome" is characterized by all of the above features, and is rare. Exposure to other antiepileptic drugs (trimethadione, phenobarbitol, carbamazepine) can produce similar anomalies.

6. Discontinuation of all medications prior to conception should be considered in women who have been seizure free for 2 or more years, although 25–40% of such women will develop a recurrence of their seizures during a subsequent pregnancy.

7. Labor and delivery is an especially susceptible time with respect to generalized tonic-clonic seizures, with occurrence in up to 4% of women with epilepsy. The reason for this is unclear, but may be related to a reduction in progesterone activity in anticipation of labor, disruption in sleep, and poor compliance with anticonvulsant medications. All medications should be continued during labor and delivery, although benzodiazepines should be used with caution in labor as they can cause maternal and neonatal depression. In most women with epilepsy, labor and delivery is uneventful.

All anticonvulsant medications cross into breast milk to some degree. The amount of transmission varies with the drug (2% for valproic acid; 30–45% for phenytoin, phenobarbital, and carbamazepine; 90% for ethosuximide). However, the use of such medications is not a contraindication to breastfeeding.

8. Seizures can cause maternal hypoxemia with resultant fetal injury, and inpatient care may be required to control convulsions. The aim of therapy is to control convulsions with a single agent using the lowest possible dose, but multiple agents may be required in refractory cases.

9. Status epilepticus refers to repeated convulsions with no intervals of consciousness. It is a medical emergency for both mother and fetus. The management is as for nonpregnant women: maintain maternal vital functions, control convulsions, and prevent subsequent seizures. A transient fetal bradycardia is common in this setting, and every effort should be made to resuscitate the fetus *in utero* before making a decision about delivery. Prolonged seizure activity (>10 min) may be associated with placental abruption.

18 Systemic Lupus Erythematosus

Consider the diagnosis of SLE[1]
- Take a detailed history, perform a physical examination, and perform relevant immunologic tests[2]
- Understand the normal physiologic changes in the immune system during pregnancy[3]
- Consider the differential diagnosis[4]

Confirm the diagnosis
- **Consult an internist, rheumatologist, and/or hematologist**
- Be aware of the effects of pregnancy on SLE[5]
- Be aware of the effects of SLE on pregnancy[6]

First prenatal visit
- √ baseline CBC, creatinine, urinalysis, and 24-h urine collection for creatinine clearance and protein estimation
- Adjust medications as needed with appropriate consultation[7]

Low risk of adverse pregnancy events[8]
- Continue routine prenatal care
- Fetal anatomic survey at 18–22 weeks (routine fetal echo is not indicated)
- In women with anti-Ro/La antibodies, measure and document fetal heart rate at each prenatal visit
- *Consider rheumatology follow-up*
- *Serial growth scans* q 3–4 weeks starting at 24 weeks
- *Weekly fetal surveillance* from 28–32 weeks

Recommend routine induction
of labor at or after 39 weeks

High risk of adverse pregnancy events[8]
- Continue routine prenatal care
- Consider baseline chest X-ray, EKG, and ABG
- Fetal anatomic survey at 18–22 weeks (routine fetal echo is not indicated)
- Continue baseline therapy[7]
- **Regular rheumatology follow-up**
- **In women with anti-Ro/La antibodies, measure and document fetal heart rate at each prenatal visit**
- *Serial growth scans* q 3–4 weeks starting at 24 weeks
- *Weekly fetal surveillance* from 28–32 weeks
- √ for pregnancy complications, especially pre-eclampsia[6]

Consider induction of labor at or 36 weeks with
documentation of fetal lung maturity

Pediatricians at delivery to evaluate for neonatal lupus

Obstetric Clinical Algorithms: Management and Evidence. By © E.R. Norwitz, M. Belfort, G.R. Saade and H. Miller.
Published 2010 Blackwell Publishing.

1. Systemic lupus erythematosus (SLE) is a chronic inflammatory disease of unknown cause which can affect the skin, joints, kidneys, lungs, nervous system, serous membranes and/or other organs of the body. Immunologic abnormalities, especially the production of a number of antinuclear antibodies, are another prominent feature of the disease. The clinical course of SLE is variable and may be characterized by periods of remissions and chronic or acute relapses.

2. Patients with SLE are subject to myriad symptoms and signs, including a mixture of constitutional complaints (fatigue, malaise, fever, and weight loss, which can be seen in 50–100% of cases) and evidence of skin (photosensitive rash, Raynaud phenomenon, mucocutaneous lesions, alopecia), musculoskeletal (arthralgia or arthritis), gastrointestinal, and serologic involvement (serositis). Some patients have predominantly hematologic, renal or central nervous system (seizures, psychosis) manifestations. Autoantibody testing is indicated, including antinuclear antibodies (ANA), antiphospholipid antibodies (see Chapter 5), antibodies to double-stranded DNA (dsDNA), and anti-smooth muscle (sm) antibodies. Measurement of serum complement levels (total hemolytic complement (CH50), C3, and C4) may also be helpful, since hypocomplementemia is a frequent finding in active SLE. Once the diagnosis is confirmed, check maternal anti-Ro (SS-A) and anti-La (SS-B) antibodies.

3. The maternal immune system remains largely intact throughout pregnancy, and pregnant women should not be considered to be immunosuppressed. The one exception is cellular immunity, which is selectively depressed in pregnancy. As a result, pregnant women may be at increased risk for contracting some viral infections and tuberculosis. As regards the fetal immune system, fetal IgG is derived almost exclusively from the mother. Receptor-mediated transport of IgG from mother to fetus begins at 16 weeks' gestation, but the bulk of IgG is acquired in the last 4 weeks of pregnancy. As such, preterm infants have very low circulating IgG levels. IgM is not actively transported across the placenta. As such, IgM levels in the fetus accurately reflect the response of the fetal immune system to infection. B lymphocytes appear in the fetal liver by 9 weeks and in the blood and spleen by 12 weeks. T cells leave the fetal thymus at around 14 weeks. The fetus does not acquire much IgG (passive immunity) from colostrum, although IgA in breast milk may protect against some enteric infections.

4. The differential diagnosis of SLE is extensive and depends on the dominant clinical manifestations. Other rheumatologic conditions should be considered, including Sjögren syndrome and rheumatoid arthritis.

5. Systemic lupus erythematosus does not generally worsen in pregnancy. The frequency of exacerbations (or persistently active disease) is dependent in large part on the state of disease activity at the time of conception and on continuation of medications.

6. Women with SLE are more likely to have pregnancy complications, including spontaneous abortion, gestational hypertension/pre-eclampsia, preterm birth, cesarean delivery, postpartum hemorrhage, venous thromboembolic disorders (DVT, PE), intrauterine growth restriction (IUGR), and stillbirths and neonatal deaths. Maternal anti-Ro (SS-A) and anti-La (SS-B) antibodies are associated with complete fetal heart block in 5–10% of cases. SLE does not confer risks for other identifiable congenital abnormalities.

7. Corticosteroids, antimalarials (chloroquine, hydroxychloroquine), antihypertensives (with the exception of angiotensin-converting enzyme (ACE) inhibitors), and select cytotoxic agents (azathioprine) are safe in pregnancy. Cyclophosphamide, cyclosporine, and penicillamine may have adverse fetal effects, but may be used if indicated. Nonsteroidal anti-inflammatory drugs (NSAID), mycophenolate, methotrexate, warfarin, anti-TNF-α agents, B-cell targeted antibodies (rituximab), and T-/B-cell co-stimulation blockers (abatacept) are best avoided in pregnancy, either because they have well-documented adverse effects or because there is little data on their safety in pregnancy.

8. A number of characteristics are associated with high maternal and fetal risk, including: poorly controlled hypertension; severe pulmonary hypertension (mean pressure >50 mmHg); restrictive lung disease (forced vital capacity <1 L); cardiac failure; chronic renal failure (creatinine >2.8 mg/dL); history of severe pre-eclampsia; stroke within the previous 6 months; and severe lupus flare within the previous 6 months.

19 Thrombocytopenia

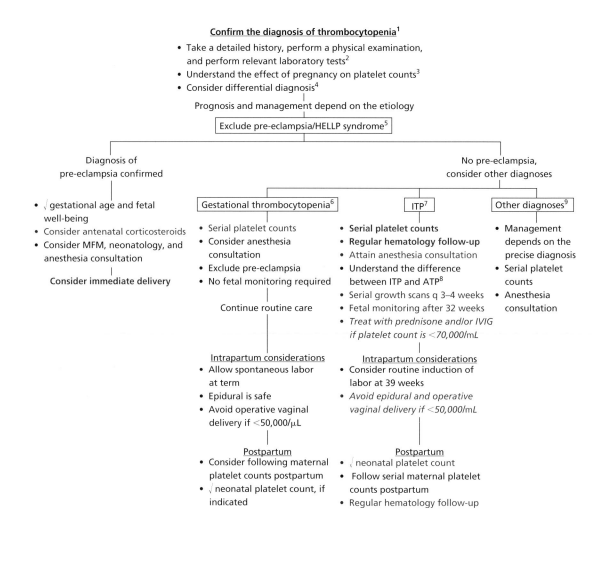

Confirm the diagnosis of thrombocytopenia[1]
- Take a detailed history, perform a physical examination, and perform relevant laboratory tests[2]
- Understand the effect of pregnancy on platelet counts[3]
- Consider differential diagnosis[4]

Prognosis and management depend on the etiology

Exclude pre-eclampsia/HELLP syndrome[5]

Diagnosis of pre-eclampsia confirmed
- √ gestational age and fetal well-being
- Consider antenatal corticosteroids
- Consider MFM, neonatology, and anesthesia consultation

Consider immediate delivery

No pre-eclampsia, consider other diagnoses

Gestational thrombocytopenia[6]
- Serial platelet counts
- Consider anesthesia consultation
- Exclude pre-eclampsia
- No fetal monitoring required

Continue routine care

Intrapartum considerations
- Allow spontaneous labor at term
- Epidural is safe
- Avoid operative vaginal delivery if <50,000/μL

Postpartum
- Consider following maternal platelet counts postpartum
- √ neonatal platelet count, if indicated

ITP[7]
- **Serial platelet counts**
- **Regular hematology follow-up**
- Attain anesthesia consultation
- Understand the difference between ITP and ATP[8]
- Serial growth scans q 3–4 weeks
- Fetal monitoring after 32 weeks
- *Treat with prednisone and/or IVIG if platelet count is <70,000/mL*

Intrapartum considerations
- Consider routine induction of labor at 39 weeks
- *Avoid epidural and operative vaginal delivery if <50,000/mL*

Postpartum
- √ neonatal platelet count
- Follow serial maternal platelet counts postpartum
- Regular hematology follow-up

Other diagnoses[9]
- Management depends on the precise diagnosis
- Serial platelet counts
- Anesthesia consultation

Obstetric Clinical Algorithms: Management and Evidence. By © E.R. Norwitz, M. Belfort, G.R. Saade and H. Miller.
Published 2010 Blackwell Publishing.

1. Thrombocytopenia (low platelets) complicates 5–15% of all gestations. Unlike nonpregnant women (in whom a cut-off of <150,000 platelets/μL is used), thrombocytopenia in pregnancy is defined as a circulating platelet level of <100,000/μL. Routine CBC measurements at the first prenatal visit and again in the third trimester will identify women with asymptomatic thrombocytopenia.

2. Ask about pre-existing medical and hematologic conditions, medications which can affect platelet counts (such as heparin) or bleeding time, and symptoms of excessive bleeding. Physical examination may reveal a petechial skin rash, subconjunctival hemorrhage or other evidence of excessive bleeding (bruising, leakage from intravenous sites or bleeding into joints).

3. Although platelet counts are normal in most women during uncomplicated pregnancy, the mean platelet counts of pregnant women are lower than in healthy nonpregnant women, due primarily to hemodilution. Serial platelet counts are more useful than a single measurement.

4. The differential diagnosis of thrombocytopenia in pregnancy includes gestational thrombocytopenia, immune thrombocytopenic purpura (ITP), pre-eclampsia/HELLP syndrome, coagulopathy (including consumptive coagulopathy), thrombotic thrombocytopenic purpura/hemolytic uremic syndrome (TTP/HUS), and drug-induced thrombocytopenia.

5. See Chapter 12.

6. Gestational thrombocytopenia is defined by five criteria: (i) mild and asymptomatic thrombocytopenia (platelet counts are typically >70,000/μL); (ii) no past history of thrombocytopenia (except during a previous pregnancy); (iii) occurrence during late gestation; (iv) no association with fetal thrombocytopenia (vs 10–15% neonatal thrombocytopenia in patients with ITP); and (v) spontaneous resolution after delivery. It is likely due to hemodilution alone, although an immunologic etiology cannot be definitively excluded. For both mother and infant, routine obstetric management is appropriate. Epidural anesthesia is safe in women with gestational thrombocytopenia who have platelet counts >70,000/μL. Women with documented thrombocytopenia should be followed with platelet counts to determine if spontaneous resolution occurs after delivery. The risk of neonatal bleeding complications (including intracranial hemorrhage) is extremely low. There are no long-term studies to determine whether women with gestational thrombocytopenia have a greater risk of developing ITP.

7. Immune thrombocytopenic purpura (ITP) is a maternal disease characterized by the presence of circulating antiplatelet antibodies. The distinction between gestational thrombocytopenia and ITP is largely empiric, although ITP is the more likely diagnosis if thrombocytopenia occurs early in pregnancy or if the platelet count is very low (<50,000/μL). The prognosis and management depend on the severity of the thrombocytopenia. In addition to maternal bleeding complications, IgG can cross the placenta and cause fetal thrombocytopenia. At delivery, 10% of infants born to women with ITP will have a platelet count <50,000/μL and 5% will have a count <20,000/μL. The correlation between maternal platelet counts, maternal antiplatelet antibody levels, and fetal platelet counts is poor. Daily glucocorticoid therapy should be considered if the maternal platelet count is low (<70,000/μL). Intravenous immune globulin (IVIG), plasmapharesis, and splenectomy are rarely necessary in pregnancy. Cesarean delivery has not been shown to improve perinatal outcome and should be reserved for usual obstetric indications. The old practice of percutaneous umbilical blood sampling (PUBS) at 38 weeks to determine the fetal platelet count has a mortality rate of 2%, which is greater than the risk of severe fetal/neonatal intracerebral hemorrhage (<1%), and has therefore been abandoned.

8. Alloimmune thrombocytopenia (ATP) is a condition in which maternal platelet counts are normal, but antiplatelet antibodies (usually anti-PLA1/2) cross the placenta to cause fetal thrombocytopenia and possibly intraventricular hemorrhage. ATP is analogous to Rh disease of platelets.

9. Other causes of thrombocytopenia include drug-induced thrombocytopenia, coagulopathy, and TTP/HUS. TTP/HUS is rare (1 in 25,000) and can occur at any time in pregnancy. There are no pathognomonic findings for TTP/HUS, and the diagnosis is based upon the clinician's judgment after considering the history, physical examination, and laboratory findings. TTP/HUS must be distinguished from pre-eclampsia. The primary treatment for pre-eclampsia is delivery; the primary treatment for TTP/HUS is plasma exchange, as it is in nonpregnant patients. Termination of the pregnancy is usually not required for TTP/HUS.

20 Thyroid Dysfunction

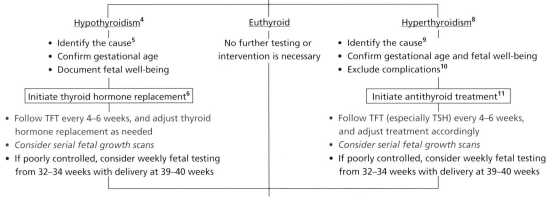

Thyroid dysfunction in pregnancy

- Be aware of physiologic changes in maternal thyroid function in pregnancy[1]
- Fetal thyroid function is independent of maternal thyroid function[2]

Confirm the diagnosis of thyroid dysfunction

- Perform a detailed history and physical examination[3]
- Check thyroid function tests (TFT)

Hypothyroidism[4]	Euthyroid	Hyperthyroidism[8]
• Identify the cause[5]	No further testing or	• Identify the cause[9]
• Confirm gestational age	intervention is necessary	• Confirm gestational age and fetal well-being
• Document fetal well-being		• Exclude complications[10]

Initiate thyroid hormone replacement[6]

- Follow TFT every 4–6 weeks, and adjust thyroid hormone replacement as needed
- *Consider serial fetal growth scans*
- If poorly controlled, consider weekly fetal testing from 32–34 weeks with delivery at 39–40 weeks

Initiate antithyroid treatment[11]

- Follow TFT (especially TSH) every 4–6 weeks, and adjust treatment accordingly
- *Consider serial fetal growth scans*
- If poorly controlled, consider weekly fetal testing from 32–34 weeks with delivery at 39–40 weeks

- **Follow closely for postpartum thyroiditis[7]**
- **Ensure adequate endocrinology follow-up**

1. Thyroid functions change in pregnancy. Levothyroxine (T_4) and L-triiodothyronine (T_3) are bound primarily to thyroxine-binding globulin (TBG) with <1% circulating as free (biologically active) hormone. T_4 is a prohormone that is converted to biologically active T_3 in peripheral tissues. High estrogen levels increase TBG production in the liver by 75–100% and stimulate TBG sialylation, which reduces hepatic clearance of T_4 and T_3. The end result is a 10–30% increase in *total* T_4 and T_3 in the maternal circulation during pregnancy, but no change in circulating thyroid stimulating hormone (TSH) or *free* T_4 and T_3.

2. <0.1% of thyroid hormone crosses the placenta. As such, fetal thyroid function is entirely independent of maternal thyroid function, although the fetus does require iodine from the maternal diet to make thyroid hormone.

Thyroid hormone can be measured in fetal blood as early as 12 weeks' gestation.

3. Symptoms and signs may suggest the diagnosis of maternal thyroid dysfunction (see below). However, as in nonpregnant patients, confirmation of maternal thyroid dysfunction in pregnancy requires thyroid function testing, specifically TSH and free T_4 and T_3. Of note, although subclinical hypothyroidism has been associated in some studies with long-term cognitive deficits in the offspring, routine screening of all pregnant women is not currently recommended.

4. *Maternal hypothyroidism* complicates 0.6% of all pregnancies. Common symptoms of thyroid hormone deficiency include fatigue, cold intolerance, weight gain, constipation,

Obstetric Clinical Algorithms: Management and Evidence. By © E.R. Norwitz, M. Belfort, G.R. Saade and H. Miller.
Published 2010 Blackwell Publishing.

myalgia, and menstrual irregularities, but such symptoms are nonspecific and are commonly attributed to normal pregnancy. A goiter is a common finding on examination. Thyroid function testing is required for a definitive diagnosis with an elevated TSH (>5.0 mU/mL) and decreased free T_4 and T_3. Measurement of circulating antithyroid antibodies is not helpful in confirming the diagnosis.

5. Causes of hypothyroidism include (i) Hashimoto thyroiditis (chronic lymphocytic thyroiditis) which is characterized by hypothyroidism, a firm goiter, and the presence of circulating antithyroglobulin or antimicrosomal antibodies. (ii) Women previously treated for hyperthyroidism by surgery or ^{131}I ablation may manifest with hypothyroidism and require thyroid hormone replacement. (iii) Infectious (suppurative) thyroiditis is characterized by fever and a painful, swollen thyroid gland. (iv) Subacute thyroiditis is similar to suppurative thyroiditis with a painful, swollen thyroid with or without fever. It is usually the result of a viral infection, and is self-limiting. (v) Iodine deficiency (rare).

6. Early treatment is essential to avoid pregnancy complications (IUGR, placental abruption, stillbirth) and impaired neonatal and childhood development (cretinism). Start levothyroxine (thyroxine) replacement at 100–150 μg daily. Follow TSH levels every 4–6 weeks and adjust dosing accordingly. Women on thyroxine prior to pregnancy should have TSH levels monitored every 4–6 weeks. Most women will need to increase their dose by 30–50% during pregnancy.

7. *Postpartum thyroiditis* complicates 4–10% of all pregnancies. The etiology is unknown, but it is likely an autoimmune phenomenon. It is characterized by a transient hyperthyroid state occurring 2–3 months postpartum (with dizziness, fatigue, weight loss, palpitations) and/or a transient hypothyroid state 4–8 months postpartum (with fatigue, weight gain, and depression). Treatment may be needed to control symptoms, but can usually be tapered within 1 year.

8. *Maternal hyperthyroidism (thyrotoxicosis)* refers to the clinical state resulting from an excess production of and exposure to thyroid hormone. It complicates 0.05–0.2% of all pregnancies. Common symptoms include anxiety, emotional lability, weakness, tremor, palpitations, heat intolerance, increased perspiration, weight loss, hyperdefecation (not diarrhea), and urinary frequency. Thyroid function testing is required for a definitive diagnosis with a depressed TSH (<0.05 mU/mL) and elevated free T_4 and T_3. The presence of circulating antithyroid antibodies alone is not sufficient to confirm the diagnosis.

9. Causes of hyperthyroidism include (i) Graves disease (>95% of all cases) due to circulating thyroid-stimulating autoantibodies. Ophthalmopathy (lid lag, lid retraction) and dermopathy (pretibial edema) are specific to Graves disease. Since IgG antibodies cross the placenta, the fetus is at risk of thyroid dysfunction. (ii) Toxic multinodular goiter. (ii) Solitary toxic thyroid nodule. (iv) Inflammation (thyroiditis) such as de Quervain thyroiditis is acute in onset with a painful goiter. (v) Hyperemesis gravidarum/ gestational trophoblastic neoplasia likely secondary to elevated levels of hCG. (vi) Metastatic follicular cell carcinoma of the thyroid. (vii) Exogenous T_4 or T_3. (viii) TSH-secreting pituitary adenoma.

10. Maternal complications of hyperthyroidism include infertility, recurrent pregnancy loss, cardiac failure (10–20%), and thyroid storm (<0.1%). Fetal complications include preterm birth, IUGR, and increased perinatal mortality.

11. Antithyroid drugs includes propylthiouracil (PTU) and carbimazole. PTU is preferred because it blocks the release of hormone from the thyroid gland and (unlike carbimazole) also blocks peripheral conversion of T_4 to T_3. Carbimazole has been associated with a rare congenital anomaly (aplasia cutis congenita). PTU treatment is initiated at 100–150 mg tid, but it can take 3–4 weeks before a clinical response is seen. Radioactive iodine to ablate the thyroid gland is absolutely contraindicated in pregnancy. Surgery is best avoided in pregnancy but, if indicated for failed medical therapy, is best performed in the second trimester. Fetal tachycardia (>160 bpm) is a sensitive index of fetal hyperthyroidism.

SECTION 3
Infectious Complications

21 Asymptomatic Bacteriuria[1]

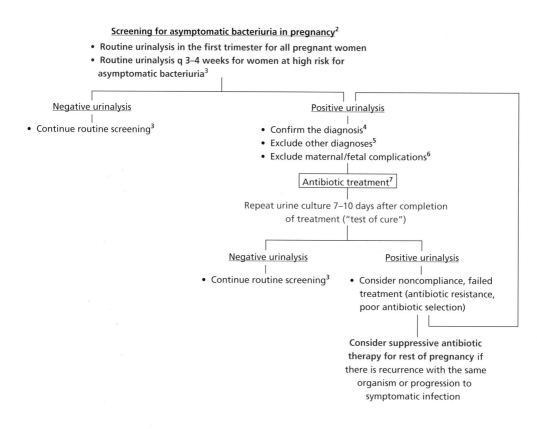

<u>Screening for asymptomatic bacteriuria in pregnancy[2]</u>
- Routine urinalysis in the first trimester for all pregnant women
- Routine urinalysis q 3–4 weeks for women at high risk for asymptomatic bacteriuria[3]

<u>Negative urinalysis</u>
- Continue routine screening[3]

<u>Positive urinalysis</u>
- Confirm the diagnosis[4]
- Exclude other diagnoses[5]
- Exclude maternal/fetal complications[6]

Antibiotic treatment[7]

Repeat urine culture 7–10 days after completion of treatment ("test of cure")

<u>Negative urinalysis</u>
- Continue routine screening[3]

<u>Positive urinalysis</u>
- Consider noncompliance, failed treatment (antibiotic resistance, poor antibiotic selection)

Consider suppressive antibiotic therapy for rest of pregnancy if there is recurrence with the same organism or progression to symptomatic infection

Obstetric Clinical Algorithms: Management and Evidence. By © E.R. Norwitz, M. Belfort, G.R. Saade and H. Miller. Published 2010 Blackwell Publishing.

1. Asymptomatic bacteriuria refers to significant bacterial colonization of the urinary tract in the absence of urinary tract symptoms. The most common pathogen is *E. coli* (65–80%). Asymptomatic bacteriuria complicates 5–10% of all pregnancies. It is not more common in pregnancy than in nonpregnant women, but is more likely to be symptomatic and progress to pyelonephritis during pregnancy.

2. Routine screening and treatment will prevent 80% of pyelonephritis in pregnancy.

3. Women at increased risk for asymptomatic bacteriuria and symptomatic urinary tract infections include those with diabetes mellitus, prior urinary tract infection in the index pregnancy, and sickle cell trait/disease.

4. While the urine dipstix can be positive for nitrates and/or leukocyte esterase, the definitive diagnosis of asymptomatic bacteriuria requires a urinalysis and urine culture demonstrating $\geq$ 100,000 CFU/mL of a single pathogenic organism in a midstream clean-catch urine specimen. Imaging studies are not indicated to confirm the diagnosis.

5. The differential diagnosis of asymptomatic bacteriuria includes contamination with lower genital tract organisms, acute cystitis, and pyelonephritis. Women with asymptomatic bacteriuria are typically asymptomatic with a benign abdominal exam. Women who are symptomatic (with complaints of frequency, urgency or dysuria) or have clinical evidence of fever or suprapubic/costovertebral angle tenderness should be diagnosed with symptomatic urinary tract infection.

6. Maternal complications include progression to symptomatic urinary infection (cystitis, pyelonephritis), urosepsis, ARDS, preterm labor, transient renal dysfunction, and anemia. Progression from asymptomatic bacteriuria to pyelonephritis in pregnancy is 13–65% if untreated, but only 2–3% if treated. Fetal complications (sepsis, low birthweight, preterm birth) are rare.

7. Antibiotic treatment should be continued for 7–10 days because of the high recurrence rate. Adequate treatment options include trimethoprim/sulfamethoxazole 160/180 mg po bid, nitrofurantoin 100 mg po bid or cephalexin 500 mg po qid. Aggressive oral hydration should also be recommended. Antibiotic therapy should be adjusted according to culture results, if indicated.

22 Urinary Tract Infection/Pyelonephritis

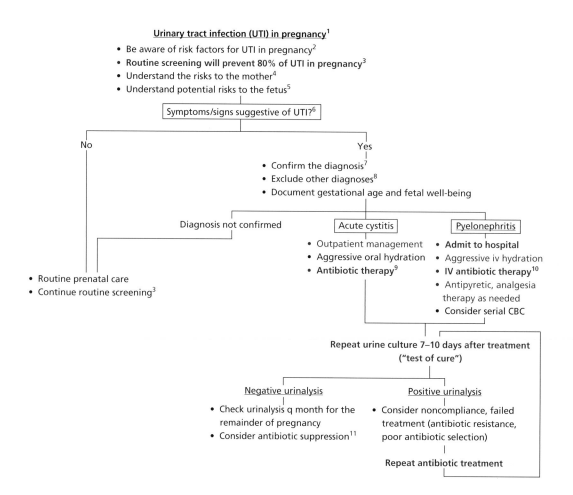

Urinary tract infection (UTI) in pregnancy[1]
- Be aware of risk factors for UTI in pregnancy[2]
- **Routine screening will prevent 80% of UTI in pregnancy[3]**
- Understand the risks to the mother[4]
- Understand potential risks to the fetus[5]

Symptoms/signs suggestive of UTI?[6]

No

Yes
- Confirm the diagnosis[7]
- Exclude other diagnoses[8]
- Document gestational age and fetal well-being

Diagnosis not confirmed

Acute cystitis
- Outpatient management
- Aggressive oral hydration
- **Antibiotic therapy[9]**

Pyelonephritis
- **Admit to hospital**
- Aggressive iv hydration
- **IV antibiotic therapy[10]**
- Antipyretic, analgesia therapy as needed
- Consider serial CBC

- Routine prenatal care
- Continue routine screening[3]

Repeat urine culture 7–10 days after treatment ("test of cure")

Negative urinalysis
- Check urinalysis q month for the remainder of pregnancy
- Consider antibiotic suppression[11]

Positive urinalysis
- Consider noncompliance, failed treatment (antibiotic resistance, poor antibiotic selection)

Repeat antibiotic treatment

Obstetric Clinical Algorithms: Management and Evidence. By © E.R. Norwitz, M. Belfort, G.R. Saade and H. Miller.
Published 2010 Blackwell Publishing.

1. Urinary tract infections (UTI) include acute cystitis and pyelonephritis, and complicate 3–4% and 1–2% of pregnancies, respectively. The most common pathogens are *Escherichia coli* (80–90%) and *Staphylococcus saprophyticus* (4–7%).

2. Risk factors for UTI in pregnancy include women with diabetes mellitus, prior UTI in the index pregnancy, urinary tract anomalies, and sickle cell trait/disease.

3. See Asymptomatic bacteriuria (Chapter 21).

4. Risks to the mother of untreated cystitis include progression to pyelonephritis. Complications of pyelonephritis include urosepsis (10–15%) leading to septic shock (1–3%), ARDS (2–8%), anemia (25–50%), transient renal dysfunction (25%), and preterm labor.

5. Potential risks to the fetus include preterm birth and low birthweight.

6. Symptoms of acute cystitis include urinary frequency, dysuria, urgency, and suprapubic pain; systemic complaints are usually absent. Physical examination may reveal suprapubic tenderness, but is usually unhelpful. Systemic symptoms of fever, chills, nausea, vomiting, and flank pain suggest a diagnosis of pyelonephritis. In such cases, there may be evidence of flank or costovertebral angle tenderness on physical examination.

7. While the urine dipstix can be positive for nitrates and/or leukocyte esterase, the definitive diagnosis of UTI requires a urinalysis and urine culture with ≥100,000 colony-forming units (CFU)/mL of a single pathogenic organism in a midstream clean-catch urine specimen. Imaging studies are not indicated to confirm the diagnosis. If the patient is febrile, send a CBC and consider blood cultures to exclude urosepsis.

8. Differential diagnosis includes contamination with lower genital tract organisms, asymptomatic bacteriuria, and lower genital tract infection (such as bacterial vaginosis or yeast infection). In the setting of pyelonephritis, consider also urosepsis, appendicitis, cholecystitis, and lower lobe pneumonia.

9. Appropriate treatment options for cystitis include trimethoprim/sulfamethoxazole 160/180 mg po bid, nitrofurantoin 100 mg po bid or cephalexin 500 mg po qid. Medications should be adjusted according to culture results. Duration of antibiotic treatment should be 3–5 days for otherwise healthy women or 7–10 days for women with concurrent chronic disease. Single-dose therapy is associated with an increased failure rate in pregnancy and is not recommended.

10. Appropriate treatment options for pyelonephritis include: (i) ampicillin 2 g q6h + gentamicin 1.5 mg/kg q8h iv; (ii) cefazolin 1 g q8h iv; (iii) ceftriaxone 12 g q24h iv/im; (iv) mezlocillin 1–3 g iv q6h; or (v) piperacillin 4 g iv q8h. Antibiotics should be continued until 24–48 hours afebrile.

11. Women who have two or more episodes of acute cystits or one or more episodes of pyelonephritis should be given suppressive antibiotic therapy (nitrofurantoin 50–100 mg po each night) for the remainder of the pregnancy and should have urine cultures checked every month until delivery.

23 Lower Genital Tract Infections

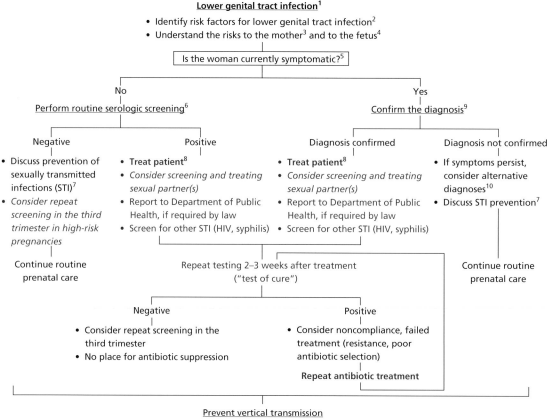

Lower genital tract infection[1]
- Identify risk factors for lower genital tract infection[2]
- Understand the risks to the mother[3] and to the fetus[4]

Is the woman currently symptomatic?[5]

No

Perform routine serologic screening[6]

Negative
- Discuss prevention of sexually transmitted infections (STI)[7]
- *Consider repeat screening in the third trimester in high-risk pregnancies*

Continue routine prenatal care

Positive
- **Treat patient[8]**
- *Consider screening and treating sexual partner(s)*
- Report to Department of Public Health, if required by law
- Screen for other STI (HIV, syphilis)

Yes

Confirm the diagnosis[9]

Diagnosis confirmed
- **Treat patient[8]**
- *Consider screening and treating sexual partner(s)*
- Report to Department of Public Health, if required by law
- Screen for other STI (HIV, syphilis)

Diagnosis not confirmed
- If symptoms persist, consider alternative diagnoses[10]
- Discuss STI prevention[7]

Continue routine prenatal care

Repeat testing 2–3 weeks after treatment ("test of cure")

Negative
- Consider repeat screening in the third trimester
- No place for antibiotic suppression

Positive
- Consider noncompliance, failed treatment (resistance, poor antibiotic selection)

Repeat antibiotic treatment

Prevent vertical transmission
- Topical treatment to all neonates at delivery[11]

1. Lower genital tract infections include: (i) bacterial vaginosis (BV), which refers to an overgrowth of commensal vaginal organisms, including *Bacteroides, Peptostreptococcus, Gardnerella vaginalis, Mycoplasma hominis,* and Enterobacteriaceae with a decrease in lactobacillus species. It is not a sexually transmitted infection (STI); (ii) trichomonas, a predominantly (but not exclusively) STI caused by *Trichomonas vaginalis*; (iii) gonorrhea, an STI caused by *Neisseria gonorrhea*; and

(iv) chlamydia, the most common STI in the United States caused by the obligate intracellular parasite *Chlamydia trachomatis*.

2. Risk factors for lower genital tract infections include multiple sexual partners, unprotected intercourse, other sexually transmitted infections, drug abuse, diabetes, unmarried status, age <20 years, a "high-risk" partner, and late/no prenatal care.

Obstetric Clinical Algorithms: Management and Evidence. By © E.R. Norwitz, M. Belfort, G.R. Saade and H. Miller.
Published 2010 Blackwell Publishing.

3. Lower genital tract infections are associated with an increased risk of preterm birth, especially if they are symptomatic. However, it is not clear that treatment abrogates this risk. As such, routine screening for lower genital tract infections is not generally recommended in either low- or high-risk pregnancies.

4. Aside from the risk of preterm birth, lower genital tract infections pose little risk to the fetus while *in utero*. They do not generally cause ascending intra-amniotic infection. If exposed at delivery, however, such infections (chlamydia, gonorrhea) can cause conjunctivitis and neonatal pneumonia.

5. Most women with lower genital tract infections are asymptomatic (especially chlamydia, gonorrhea, and BV). However, they may present with vulvar itching (pruritus), pain or burning that may be worse after menses or intercourse (due to a change in vaginal pH). A vaginal discharge and symptoms of dysuria may also be present. Gonorrhea can present with anal or pharyngeal discomfort. Systemic symptoms (low-grade fever, malaise, fatigue, nausea, abdominal pain) are rare, and should prompt a search for alternative causes. The exception is disseminated gonoccocal infection, which can present with fever, chills, small pustular skin lesions, and arthritis of the knees, wrists, and ankles.

6. Because chlamydia and gonorrhea are common, often asymptomatic, and can infect the fetus as it passes through the birth canal, all pregnant women should be screened for these two infections at their first prenatal visit. High-risk women should be screened again in the third trimester. A variety of screening tests are available, including (i) polymerase chain reaction (PCR)-based tests; (ii) antigen detection methods (such as ELISA or fluorescein-conjugated antibody test); (iii) cytologic staining; or (iv) culture-based protocols using selective culture media. ELISA is most commonly used in low-risk populations. Routine screening for BV and trichomonas is not recommended.

7. Prevention of STI includes avoidance of unprotected intercourse, routine use of barrier contraception, and stopping drug abuse.

8. Specific treatment depends on the infection: (i) for BV, clindamycin 2% cream vaginally daily × 7 days in early pregnancy and metronidazole 500 mg po bid or clindamycin 900 mg po bid × 7 days in the latter half of pregnancy (antibiotic therapy can be deferred in the first trimester if the woman is asymptomatic); (ii) for trichomonas, metronidazole 375–500 mg po bid × 7 days (alternative treatment includes metronidazole 2 g po × 1 dose or vaginal metronidazole/clotrimazole, but failure rate is higher); (iii) for gonorrhea, cefuroxime 400 mg po × 1 or ceftriaxone 125 mg IM × 1 dose (if penicillin allergic, use spectinomycin 2 g im × 1dose; quinolones are contraindicated in pregnancy; consider treating also for presumed chlamydia infection); and (iv) for chlamydia, amoxicillin 500 mg po tid × 7 days, erythromycin 500 mg po qid × 7 days or azithromycin 1 g po × 1 dose (topical treatment is inadequate).

9. Abdominal exam is typically benign. Speculum exam may reveal cervical erythema (a red, inflamed "strawberry" cervix is suggestive of chlamydia) and/or a cervicovaginal discharge ranging from thin malodorous (BV) to mucopurulent (gonorrhea, chlamydia) to foamy yellow-green with a foul "fishy" odor (trichomonas). Laboratory testing (ELISA) is required to confirm gonorrhea or chlamydia infection. Confirmation of trichomonas infection requires a wet smear of cervicovaginal discharge showing motile, flagellated, pear-shaped organisms. BV is a clinical diagnosis requiring at least two of the following criteria: wet mount positive for clue cells, decrease in lactobacilli, a positive "whiff test" (fishy odor) on mixture with potassium hydroxide, and vaginal pH >4.5.

10. Alternative diagnoses include urinary tract infection, ruptured membranes, foreign body, nonspecific cervicitis, herpes, and candidal (yeast) infection.

11. All infants should receive erythromycin ointment applied to their eyes within 1 hour of birth to prevent conjunctivitis from chlamydia or gonorrhea.

24 Group B Streptococcus[1]

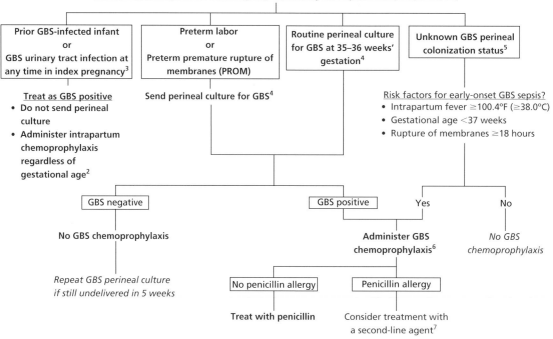

Prevention of early-onset neonatal group B β-hemolytic streptococcus (GBS) infection[2]

Prior GBS-infected infant or GBS urinary tract infection at any time in index pregnancy[3]

Treat as GBS positive
- Do not send perineal culture
- Administer intrapartum chemoprophylaxis regardless of gestational age[2]

Preterm labor or Preterm premature rupture of membranes (PROM)

Send perineal culture for GBS[4]

Routine perineal culture for GBS at 35–36 weeks' gestation[4]

Unknown GBS perineal colonization status[5]

Risk factors for early-onset GBS sepsis?
- Intrapartum fever ≥100.4°F (≥38.0°C)
- Gestational age <37 weeks
- Rupture of membranes ≥18 hours

GBS negative

No GBS chemoprophylaxis

Repeat GBS perineal culture if still undelivered in 5 weeks

GBS positive

Yes

No

Administer GBS chemoprophylaxis[6]

No GBS chemoprophylaxis

No penicillin allergy

Penicillin allergy

Treat with penicillin

Consider treatment with a second-line agent[7]

1. Group B β-h emolytic streptococcus (GBS), also known as *Streptococcus agalactiae*, is an encapsulated gram-positive coccus that colonizes the gastrointestinal and lower genital tracts of 20% (range 15–40%) of pregnant women. It is not a sexually transmitted infection. Although women whose genital tracts are colonized with GBS are typically asymptomatic, 50% of fetuses passing through a colonized birth canal will themselves be colonized with GBS and some will develop infection (also known as invasive GBS disease).

2. GBS is the most common cause of bacterial infection in the first 90 days of life. Two clinically distinct neonatal GBS infections have been identified.
- *Early-onset neonatal GBS infection* (80% of all GBS infection) results from GBS transmission during labor or delivery. It is characterized by signs of serious infection (respiratory distress, apnea, pneumonia or septic shock) within 1 week of delivery, although it presents most often within 6–12 hours of birth. The mortality rate is 5–25% and surviving infants frequently exhibit neurologic sequelae. The overall rate of early-onset neonatal GBS infection is 1–3 per 1000 livebirths, but is increased to 10 per 1000 deliveries in women colonized with GBS and may be as high as 40–50 per 1000 preterm births. This infection can be effectively prevented by intrapartum antibiotic chemoprophylaxis.
- *Late-onset neonatal GBS infection* (20%) is a hospital- (nosocomial) or community-acquired infection. It presents more than a week after birth, usually as meningitis. The mortality rate is lower than for early-onset disease, but neurologic sequelae are equally common. This

---

Obstetric Clinical Algorithms: Management and Evidence. By © E.R. Norwitz, M. Belfort, G.R. Saade and H. Miller.
Published 2010 Blackwell Publishing.

infection cannot be effectively prevented by intrapartum antibiotic chemoprophylaxis.

3. Women who have had a prior infant affected with early-onset GBS infection (not simply GBS colonization in a prior pregnancy) or a GBS urinary tract infection in the index pregnancy have a high perineal colonization rate at delivery. As such, they should be regarded as GBS positive and should all receive intrapartum chemoprophylaxis. It is not necessary to check a routine GBS perineal culture in such women.

4. The Centers for Disease Control and Prevention (CDC) in the United States recommends that all pregnant women have a perineal culture at 35–36 weeks' gestation. Although GBS colonizes the lower genital tract of 20% of pregnant women at any one time, it is not the same 20% of women throughout pregnancy with an 8–10% crossover of GBS carrier status each trimester. This is why determination of GBS carrier status cannot be done at the first prenatal visit. GBS colonization increases as one moves from the cervix to the introitus. As such, the GBS culture should be taken by swabbing the lower vagina, perineum and peri-anal area (not the cervix) and the swab should be placed briefly into the anal canal. A speculum should not be used. This perineal culture should be inoculated into selective broth media (either Todd-Hewitt broth or selective blood agar), stored at room temperature, and transported to the laboratory ideally within 8 hours of collection. Results should be available within 48 hours. Cultures sent at 35–36 weeks are reliable for 5 weeks and have been shown to accurately reflect GBS carrier status at delivery. Rapid screening tests for GBS carrier status in labor have been developed but are more difficult to perform, are not available in all hospitals at all times, and have a poor sensitivity in identifying women with light (low-level) GBS colonization.

5. This group includes women presenting with preterm labor or preterm PROM prior to routine GBS perineal culture as well as women at term who did not have a routine GBS culture sent. The management of such women depends on the presence or absence of a series of risks

factors (listed above). Reliance on a risk factor-based protocol (as in the UK) results in treatment of 20–25% of women in labor with prevention of 65–70% of early-onset GBS disease. The culture-based protocol (as recommended by CDC in the US) results in treatment of 15–20% of women in labor with prevention of 70–80% of early-onset GBS disease.

6. A number of strategies have been developed to prevent early-onset neonatal GBS infection. Intrapartum, but not antepartum, antibiotic chemoprophylaxis can prevent early-onset GBS infection in GBS-positive women. Penicillin G (5 million units iv followed by 2.5 million units every 4 hours) is the treatment of choice. Ampicillin (2 g iv load followed by 1 g every 4 hours) is an alternative prophylactic regimen, but is not recommended because it has a wider spectrum of action and is therefore more likely to cause antibiotic resistance. To date, there have been no cases of GBS resistance to penicillin or ampicillin. A minimum of 4 hours of antibiotic chemoprophylaxis is recommended. Delivery prior to 1 completed hour of chemoprophylaxis may be associated with a higher incidence of early-onset neonatal GBS infection. Antibiotics should be continued until delivery is complete. Only women with chorioamnionitis require antibiotic treatment beyond delivery.

7. A number of second-line antibiotics have been recommended for GBS chemoprophylaxis in women who are allergic to penicillin, including clindamycin (900 mg iv every 8 hours), erythromycin (500 mg iv every 6 hours), a second-generation cephalosporin (such as cefazolin 2 g iv followed by 1 g every 8 hours), and vancomycin (1 g every 12 hours). Approximately 20–30% of GBS isolates are resistant to erythromycin and 10–20% are resistant to clindamycin, and these rates appear to be increasing. In GBS-positive women who have a history of severe penicillin allergy (e.g. bronchospasm, angioedema, hypotension or shock within 30 minutes of drug administration), antimicrobial susceptibility of the GBS isolates should be tested. If resistance to erythromycin and clindamycin is documented, vancomycin should be administered. An alternative approach is to perform penicillin skin testing in such women, but this is rarely done.

25 Hepatitis B[1]

- Identify risk factors for hepatitis B virus (HBV) infection[2]
- Understand the risks to the mother[3]
- Understand potential risks to the fetus[4]

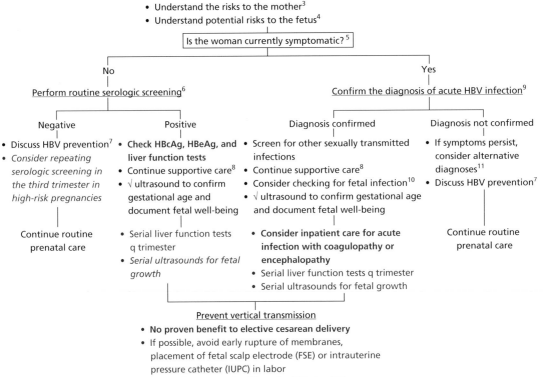

| Is the woman currently symptomatic?[5] |

No

Perform routine serologic screening[6]

Negative

- Discuss HBV prevention[7]
- *Consider repeating serologic screening in the third trimester in high-risk pregnancies*

Continue routine prenatal care

Positive

- **Check HBcAg, HBeAg, and liver function tests**
- Continue supportive care[8]
- √ ultrasound to confirm gestational age and document fetal well-being

- Serial liver function tests q trimester
- *Serial ultrasounds for fetal growth*

Yes

Confirm the diagnosis of acute HBV infection[9]

Diagnosis confirmed

- Screen for other sexually transmitted infections
- Continue supportive care[8]
- Consider checking for fetal infection[10]
- √ ultrasound to confirm gestational age and document fetal well-being

- **Consider inpatient care for acute infection with coagulopathy or encephalopathy**
- Serial liver function tests q trimester
- Serial ultrasounds for fetal growth

Diagnosis not confirmed

- If symptoms persist, consider alternative diagnoses[11]
- Discuss HBV prevention[7]

Continue routine prenatal care

Prevent vertical transmission
- **No proven benefit to elective cesarean delivery**
- If possible, avoid early rupture of membranes, placement of fetal scalp electrode (FSE) or intrauterine pressure catheter (IUPC) in labor
- **Exposed neonates should receive HBIg by 12 hours of life and the hepatitis B vaccine by 6 months**
- **Breastfeeding is not contraindicated**

Obstetric Clinical Algorithms: Management and Evidence. By © E.R. Norwitz, M. Belfort, G.R. Saade and H. Miller. Published 2010 Blackwell Publishing.

1. Viral hepatitis is caused by members of the hepatitis family of small DNA viruses. Approximately 80–85% of individuals infected with hepatitis B virus (HBV) clear the infection and develop lifelong protective immunity as evidenced by the presence of anti-hepatitis B surface antibodies (HBsAb); 10–15% remain chronically infected with detectable hepatitis B surface antigen (HBsAg) but have normal hepatic function; and 5–10% are chronically infected with persistent viral replication, elevated liver function tests, and measurable HBeAg expression (a marker of high infectivity). Acute hepatitis B occurs in 1 in 1000 pregnancies, and chronic hepatitis B is seen in 10 in 1000 pregnancies.

2. Risk factors for HBV infection include multiple sexual partners, household or occupational exposure (especially working in a hemodialysis unit), intravenous drug abuse, prior blood transfusion, and chronic hospitalization.

3. Maternal short-term complications include right upper quadrant pain, jaundice, elevated liver function tests, and (rarely) coagulopathy and encephalopathy. Serious long-term complications include cirrhosis and hepatocellular carcinoma.

4. The risk to the fetus of acquiring HBV infection is related primarily to two factors: (i) gestational age (10% risk if infected in the first trimester versus 90% if infected in the third trimester) and (ii) maternal infectivity status (10–20% if HBsAg positive only versus 90% if HBsAg and HBeAg positive). Every effort should be made to avoid amniocentesis.

5. Women with acute HBV infection are often asymptomatic. Symptoms may include low-grade fever, malaise, fatigue, nausea, abdominal pain, and jaundice.

6. Serologic screening is recommended for all pregnant women at their first prenatal visit regardless of their risk status. The clinically relevant antigens include: (i) surface antigen (HBsAg), which is found on the viral surface and free in maternal serum; (ii) core antigen (HBcAg), which is found in hepatocytes; and (iii) envelope antigen (HBeAg), which is only expressed in the setting of a high viral load and is a marker of high infectivity. Routine serologic screening includes HBsAg only. If the HBsAg screen is positive, then HBcAg and HBeAg serology should be sent along with liver function tests (transaminase levels, bilirubin) and coagulation profile. There is no place for imaging studies to confirm the diagnosis of viral hepatitis, although a right upper quadrant ultrasound may be useful to exclude other diagnoses (such as gallbladder disease).

7. Prevention of HBV infection includes avoidance of unprotected intercourse, routine use of barrier contraception, and stopping iv drug abuse. If an exposure is documented, hepatitis B immunoglobulin (HBIg) 0.06 mL/kg im should be administered with 12 hours, and the hepatitis B vaccine should be offered (two injections 6 months apart).

8. The management of maternal HBV infection is primarily supportive. Antiviral treatment with interferon-α may be recommended in nonpregnant women with chronic hepatitis, but is contraindicated in pregnancy. There is no effective treatment for HBV infection in pregnancy.

9. Physical examination is often unhelpful, but may show evidence of jaundice or abdominal tenderness. Maternal hepatitis B infection is typically confirmed by serologic testing.

10. Fetal infection can be confirmed by detection of viral particles or DNA in fetal serum, amniotic fluid or placental tissues; however, invasive prenatal testing is not routinely recommended.

11. Differential diagnosis includes other viral hepatitis infections (such as hepatitis A, C, and D), cytomegalovirus hepatitis, pancreatitis, gallbladder disease, cholestasis of pregnancy, severe pre-eclampsia/HELLP (hemolysis, elevated liver enzymes, low platelets) syndrome, and acute fatty liver of pregnancy.

26 Herpes Simplex Virus[1]

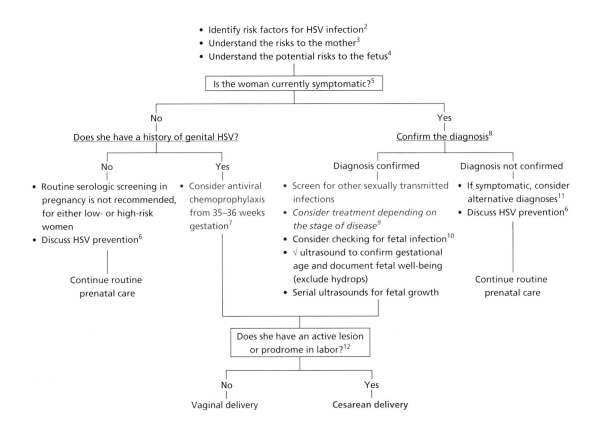

- Identify risk factors for HSV infection[2]
- Understand the risks to the mother[3]
- Understand the potential risks to the fetus[4]

Is the woman currently symptomatic?[5]

No
Does she have a history of genital HSV?

    No
- Routine serologic screening in pregnancy is not recommended, for either low- or high-risk women
- Discuss HSV prevention[6]

Continue routine prenatal care

    Yes
- Consider antiviral chemoprophylaxis from 35–36 weeks gestation[7]

Yes
Confirm the diagnosis[8]

    Diagnosis confirmed
- Screen for other sexually transmitted infections
- *Consider treatment depending on the stage of disease[9]*
- Consider checking for fetal infection[10]
- √ ultrasound to confirm gestational age and document fetal well-being (exclude hydrops)
- Serial ultrasounds for fetal growth

    Diagnosis not confirmed
- If symptomatic, consider alternative diagnoses[11]
- Discuss HSV prevention[6]

Continue routine prenatal care

Does she have an active lesion or prodrome in labor?[12]

    No
Vaginal delivery

    Yes
Cesarean delivery

Obstetric Clinical Algorithms: Management and Evidence. By © E.R. Norwitz, M. Belfort, G.R. Saade and H. Miller.
Published 2010 Blackwell Publishing.

1. Herpes simplex virus is caused by members of the Herpesviridae family of DNA viruses. There are two major serotypes: (i) HSV-1 which causes conjunctivitis, stomatitis, and gingivitis as well as 20% of genital infections; and (ii) HSV-2 which accounts for 80% of genital infections. It is the most common viral pathogen in the United States with over 45 million people infected and more than 500,000 new cases annually.

2. Risk factors include multiple sexual partners, unprotected intercourse, multiparity, other sexually transmitted infections, a history of recent exposure to HSV or intercourse with an HSV-positive partner, and history of prior HSV infection.

3. Maternal complications include localized erythema, swelling, and pain. Serious complications such as hepatitis, encephalitis, and death are rare.

4. There are 1500–2000 cases of neonatal HSV infection in the United States annually, and most are due to HSV-2. First-episode primary infection leads to a viremia and an increased risk of vertical transmission; however, *in utero* HSV infection is rare. Most neonatal infections result from contact with infected secretions at the time of vaginal delivery. Indeed, neonatal disease occurs in 30–60% of infants exposed to HSV at vaginal delivery. Recurrent HSV is not associated with viremia; as such, the fetus is not at risk if the fetal membranes remain intact and there is no labor. If the fetus is infected *in utero*, complications may include preterm birth, intrauterine fetal demise or neonatal mortality (15–60%), localized infection (skin, eye, mouth, CNS), or disseminated HSV.

5. Symptoms depend on the stage of the disease
- First-episode primary infection refers to the first clinical presentation in the absence of circulating anti-HSV IgG. Typical symptoms include painful vesicles on the vulva, vagina, and/or cervix that develop 2–14 days after exposure along with tender adenopathy and systemic symptoms (low-grade fever, malaise) in two-thirds of cases. The lesions resolve spontaneously in 3–4 weeks without treatment.
- First-episode nonprimary infection refers to the first clinical presentation but in the presence of anti-HSV IgG, suggesting evidence of prior infection.
- Recurrent infection refers to reactivation of dormant virus, and symptoms are generally less severe with no systemic features.

6. Prevention of HSV includes avoiding contact with infected persons and the routine use of barrier contraception. There is no vaccine or immune globulin available. Of note, anti-HSV-1 IgG does not prevent primary infection with HSV-2, and vice versa.

7. Antiviral chemoprophylaxis starting at 35–36 weeks' gestation is recommended for women at risk of viral shedding at delivery to decrease the likelihood of a lesion in labor requiring cesarean delivery. Whether this decreases the rate of neonatal infection is not known.

8. Maternal HSV infection can be confirmed by viral isolation from vesicular fluid or infected tissues, but problems with specimen sampling and transportation limit the sensitivity to 60–70%. Serologic testing is often performed, but is of limited utility. Such testing does not easily distinguish between anti-HSV-1 and anti-HSV-2 antibodies, and in excess of 30% of all pregnant women have anti-HSV-2 IgG.

9. The management of maternal HSV infection is primarily supportive. Antiviral treatment of first-episode primary HSV can decrease the severity and duration of symptoms in the mother, but does not prevent fetal infection. Acyclovir is the treatment of choice; alternatives include valacyclovir and famciclovir. Topical is less effective than oral treatment and is therefore not recommended. Disseminated disease should be treated with iv acyclovir in an ICU setting. It is unclear whether antiviral treatment decreases the severity or duration of symptoms in recurrent HSV infections, although it may abort an outbreak if given during the clinical prodrome or within 1 day of the onset of lesions.

10. Fetal infection can be confirmed by detection of viral particles or DNA in fetal serum, amniotic fluid or placental tissues; however, invasive prenatal testing is not routinely recommended.

11. Differential diagnosis includes other herpesvirus infections, such as varicella zoster.

12. To prevent vertical transmission, cesarean delivery should be recommended for all women with an active genital lesion or clinical prodrome in labor. Due to the low yield of viral cultures and poor correlation between culture and asymptomatic viral shedding in labor, screening for viral shedding in labor is not recommended.

27 Human Immunodeficiency Virus[1]

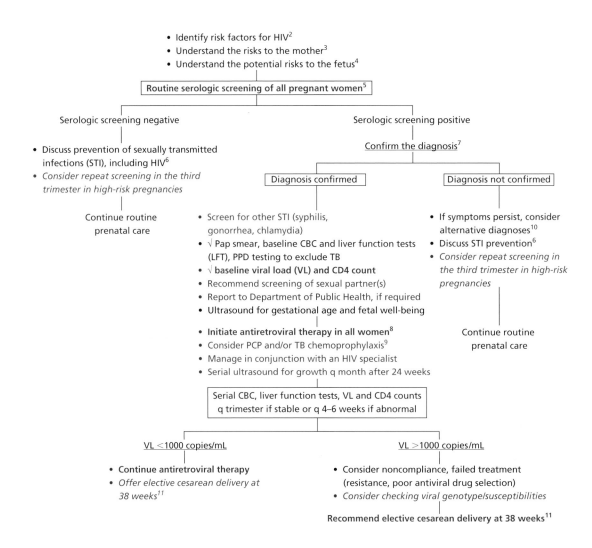

- Identify risk factors for HIV[2]
- Understand the risks to the mother[3]
- Understand the potential risks to the fetus[4]

Routine serologic screening of all pregnant women[5]

Serologic screening negative

- Discuss prevention of sexually transmitted infections (STI), including HIV[6]
- *Consider repeat screening in the third trimester in high-risk pregnancies*

Continue routine prenatal care

Serologic screening positive

Confirm the diagnosis[7]

Diagnosis confirmed

- Screen for other STI (syphilis, gonorrhea, chlamydia)
- √ Pap smear, baseline CBC and liver function tests (LFT), PPD testing to exclude TB
- √ **baseline viral load (VL) and CD4 count**
- Recommend screening of sexual partner(s)
- Report to Department of Public Health, if required
- Ultrasound for gestational age and fetal well-being

- **Initiate antiretroviral therapy in all women[8]**
- Consider PCP and/or TB chemoprophylaxis[9]
- Manage in conjunction with an HIV specialist
- Serial ultrasound for growth q month after 24 weeks

Serial CBC, liver function tests, VL and CD4 counts q trimester if stable or q 4–6 weeks if abnormal

VL <1000 copies/mL

- **Continue antiretroviral therapy**
- *Offer elective cesarean delivery at 38 weeks[11]*

VL >1000 copies/mL

- Consider noncompliance, failed treatment (resistance, poor antiviral drug selection)
- *Consider checking viral genotype/susceptibilities*

Recommend elective cesarean delivery at 38 weeks[11]

Diagnosis not confirmed

- If symptoms persist, consider alternative diagnoses[10]
- Discuss STI prevention[6]
- *Consider repeat screening in the third trimester in high-risk pregnancies*

Continue routine prenatal care

Obstetric Clinical Algorithms: Management and Evidence. By © E.R. Norwitz, M. Belfort, G.R. Saade and H. Miller.
Published 2010 Blackwell Publishing.

1. Human innumodeficiency virus is a single-stranded DNA virus that causes AIDS. In women, it is primarily (although not exclusively) a sexually transmitted infection (STI) acquired through heterosexual intercourse. It can also be acquired through blood transfusion, intravenous drug abuse or transplacental infection (vertical transmission). Once acquired, it cannot be eradicated.

2. Risk factors for HIV include prostitution/multiple sexual partners, unprotected intercourse, other STI, drug abuse, HIV-positive/bisexual partner, late/no prenatal care, new immigrant from a high-prevalence area (such as Africa), and a prior blood transfusion (especially before 1985).

3. Human innumodeficiency virus causes AIDS. Pregnancy does not increase progression to AIDS. In pregnancy, HIV infection is associated with an increased risk of preterm premature rupture of membranes (PROM) and preterm birth.

4. The major risk to the fetus is vertical transmission. HIV-positive infants may develop AIDS with a high mortality rate. Baseline rates of vertical transmission without treatment range from 25% to 33%. The risk appears to be highest during labor and delivery. Zidovudine (AZT) administration to the mother throughout pregnancy and during labor, and to the neonate for the first 6 weeks of life has been shown to decrease vertical transmission to 8%. Vertical transmission appears to be related to the circulating viral load (VL). If the circulating VL is less than assay (i.e. <50 copies/mL), the risk of vertical transmission decreases to <2%.

5. A history of STI, opportunistic infections (such as *Pneumocystis carinii* pneumonia (PCP)) or cervical dysplasia/cancer may suggest the diagnosis of HIV. Physical examination is usually unhelpful, but may identify nonspecific features (weight loss, skin lesions) or evidence of thrush, vaginitis, cervical lesion or generalized lymphadenopathy. However, most pregnant women with HIV are asymptomatic with no identifiable risk factors. This observation, along with the fact that treatment is now available to effectively prevent vertical transmission, mandates that all pregnant women be screened for HIV at their first prenatal visit. Maternal serum enzyme-linked immunosorbent assay (ELISA) is the most common screening test.

6. Prevention of HIV includes avoidance of unprotected intercourse, routine use of barrier contraception, and stopping drug abuse/needle sharing. Needle exchange programs have been shown to be effective in preventing HIV infection.

7. Confirmation of the diagnosis requires repeat ELISA and confirmatory HIV Western blot analysis.

8. Nonpregnant HIV-positive women with an undetectable VL do not need treatment. However, HIV-positive women should all be treated in pregnancy regardless of VL to prevent vertical transmission. Monotherapy is discouraged, because of the rapid emergence of resistance. Multidrug highly-active antiretroviral therapy (HAART) is recommended with nucleoside analog reverse transcriptase inhibitors (AZT, DDI, 3TC, D4T), protease inhibitors (indinavir, nelfinavir, ritonivir, sequanavir), and/or other drugs (nivaripine, delacirone, etacirenz). Treatment should include AZT since it is best proven to prevent vertical transmission. Women should be followed closely for drug side-effects (such as rash, bone marrow depression, and liver dysfunction).

9. If CD4 count is <200 cells/mm^3, PCP chemoprophylaxis (bactrim, inhaled pentamidine) is indicated. If CD4 count is <50 cells/mm^3, administer TB prophylaxis.

10. Alternative diagnoses include, among others, viral hepatitis, pneumonia, and anorexia.

11. In women with an elevated VL (>1000 copies/mL), elective cesarean delivery at or after 38–0/7 weeks can decrease vertical transmission to <1% (range 0–2%). Amniocentesis for fetal lung maturity testing is not required. However, once there is rupture of membranes or labor, the protective effect seems to disappear. There is no proven benefit to elective cesarean if the VL is <1000 copies/mL, although it would be reasonable to discuss mode of delivery with all HIV-positive women. If a vaginal delivery is planned, every effort should be made to avoid early amniotomy, prolonged rupture of membranes, and fetal scalp electrode placement.

28 Parvovirus B19[1]

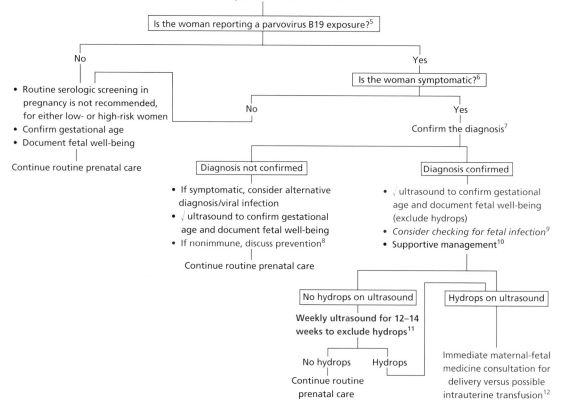

- Identify risk factors for parvovirus B19 infection[2]
- Understand the risks to the mother[3]
- Understand the potential risks to the fetus[4]

Is the woman reporting a parvovirus B19 exposure?[5]

No

- Routine serologic screening in pregnancy is not recommended, for either low- or high-risk women
- Confirm gestational age
- Document fetal well-being

Continue routine prenatal care

Yes

Is the woman symptomatic?[6]

No

Yes

Confirm the diagnosis[7]

Diagnosis not confirmed

- If symptomatic, consider alternative diagnosis/viral infection
- √ ultrasound to confirm gestational age and document fetal well-being
- If nonimmune, discuss prevention[8]

Continue routine prenatal care

Diagnosis confirmed

- √ ultrasound to confirm gestational age and document fetal well-being (exclude hydrops)
- *Consider checking for fetal infection[9]*
- Supportive management[10]

No hydrops on ultrasound

Weekly ultrasound for 12–14 weeks to exclude hydrops[11]

No hydrops

Continue routine prenatal care

Hydrops

Hydrops on ultrasound

Immediate maternal-fetal medicine consultation for delivery versus possible intrauterine transfusion[12]

Obstetric Clinical Algorithms: Management and Evidence. By © E.R. Norwitz, M. Belfort, G.R. Saade and H. Miller.
Published 2010 Blackwell Publishing.

1. Parvovirus B19 is a single-stranded DNA virus that causes fifth disease (erythema infectiosum). It is transmission by hand-to-mouth contact and respiratory secretions. The incubation period is 5–10 days although the infectious period is usually past once clinical manifestations are present.

2. Risk factors include frequent contact with children aged 5–18 years old in the home or in the workplace, professions which have regular contact with young children (such as teachers, daycare providers), Caucasian ethnicity, and age <30 years. Nonimmune fetal hydrops due to acute parvovirus B19 infection does not recur in subsequent pregnancies so a history of such an event should be regarded as protective.

3. Fifth disease is a common, self-limiting illness of childhood presenting with a reticular facial and truncal rash, mild upper respiratory tract symptoms, and a low-grade fever. Adults with fifth disease may present with a self-limiting arthropathy and, rarely, can develop a transient aplastic crisis and cardiac failure.

4. Transplacental passage of parvovirus B19 is high (33%), but the risk of fetal morbidity and mortality is low, estimated at 3% for household contact and <1% for school contact. Serious fetal sequelae usually occur with infection prior to 20 weeks' gestation, and may include anemia (due to parvovirus-induced bone marrow suppression), nonimmune hydrops (associated with a fetal hematocrit <15% – normal is approximately 50%), stillbirth, and spontaneous abortion. If the fetus survives, its long-term development appears to be normal. Of note, parvovirus B19 is not a teratogen, and exposure in early pregnancy has not been associated with any structural defects.

5. Approximately 40–50% of reproductive-age women have not previously been exposed to parvovirus B19. In susceptible women, exposure results in seroconversion in 50–70% of cases if the contact is household member and in 20% of cases if the exposure occurs at school.

6. Symptoms/signs may include a low-grade fever, joint pains, and a characteristic "slapped-cheek" facial rash.

7. Maternal parvovirus B19 infection can be confirmed by serologic testing or, less commonly, direct visualization of viral particles in infected tissues. Positive IgM or a fourfold increase in IgG titers over a period of 4–6 weeks is diagnostic of acute parvovirus B19 infection. Anti-parvovirus B19 IgM persists only for a few months, whereas IgG persists for life.

8. If a woman is known to be nonimmune, she should be counseled to avoid exposure if possible. There is no vaccine or immune globulin available.

9. Fetal infection can be confirmed by detection of viral particles or DNA in fetal serum, amniotic fluid or placental tissues; however, invasive prenatal testing is not routinely recommended.

10. The management of maternal parvovirus B19 infection is primarily supportive. There is no effective treatment and no vaccine.

11. In pregnancies with confirmed maternal parvovirus B19 infection, weekly ultrasound surveillance for 12–14 weeks is indicated to watch for the development of nonimmune hydrops. Fetal hydrops results from severe anemia (fetal hematocrit <15%) due to parvovirus-induced bone marrow suppression. After 14 weeks, the likelihood of this event is minimal and surveillance can be discontinued. Ultrasound examination should include middle cerebral artery (MCA) peak velocity measurement to identify fetuses with anemia.

12. Should hydrops develop, management options are limited to either immediate delivery if the gestational age is favorable (>34–36 weeks) or percutaneous umbilical blood sampling (PUBS) to confirm the diagnosis, to exclude other causes of nonimmune hydrops, and possibly to perform an intrauterine transfusion (IUT) to correct the anemia and reverse the hydropic changes. Serial (weekly) IUT may be required until the parvovirus infection resolves.

29 Syphilis

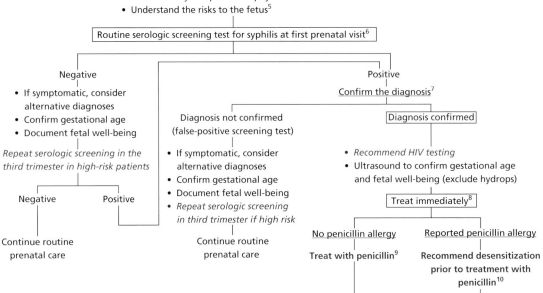

Screening for syphilis[1]
- Identify risk factors for syphilis[2]
- Be aware of the different stages of syphilis[3]
- Take a history and perform a physical examination[4]
- Understand the risks to the fetus[5]

Routine serologic screening test for syphilis at first prenatal visit[6]

Negative
- If symptomatic, consider alternative diagnoses
- Confirm gestational age
- Document fetal well-being

Repeat serologic screening in the third trimester in high-risk patients

Negative | Positive

Continue routine prenatal care

Positive
Confirm the diagnosis[7]

Diagnosis not confirmed (false-positive screening test)
- If symptomatic, consider alternative diagnoses
- Confirm gestational age
- Document fetal well-being
- *Repeat serologic screening in third trimester if high risk*

Continue routine prenatal care

Diagnosis confirmed
- *Recommend HIV testing*
- Ultrasound to confirm gestational age and fetal well-being (exclude hydrops)

Treat immediately[8]

No penicillin allergy
Treat with penicillin[9]

Reported penicillin allergy
Recommend desensitization prior to treatment with penicillin[10]

Nontreponemal antibody serologic titers (VDRL, RPR) should be checked at 1, 3, 6, 12, and 24 months after treatment[11]

1. Syphilis is a chronic infection caused by the spirochete *Treponema pallidum*. It is sexually acquired (except for cases of vertical transmission) with an incubation period of 10–90 days (average 21 days). If untreated in pregnancy, there is a high risk of fetal infection.

2. Risk factors include sexual promiscuity, illicit drug use, HIV, no prenatal care, poor socio-economic status, black or Hispanic ethnicity, and age <25 years.

3. Early syphilis (<1 year) includes primary, secondary, and early latent. Latent syphilis refers to asymptomatic infection with positive serology and no physical findings. It is divided

into early (<1 year) and late latent (>1 year). Tertiary syphilis occurs after early or latent syphilis, and typically involves the central nervous system (CNS), cardiovascular system, or skin and subcutaneous tissues. It can arise as soon as 1 year after initial infection or up to 25–30 years later.

4. History should include questions about risk factors (above). Clinical manifestations depend on the stage of the disease, and are not altered by pregnancy.

- *Primary syphilis* is characterized by a papule at the site of inoculation, which ulcerates to produce the classic painless chancer with a raised, indurated margin and

Obstetric Clinical Algorithms: Management and Evidence. By © E.R. Norwitz, M. Belfort, G.R. Saade and H. Miller.
Published 2010 Blackwell Publishing.

regional lymphadenopathy. Chancer heals spontaneously in 3–6 weeks even in the absence of treatment.

- *Secondary syphilis* is a disseminated systemic process that begins 6 weeks to 6 months after the chancer in 25% of untreated patients. Findings may include a generalized maculopapular skin rash (involving the palms, soles, and mucous membranes), generalized lymphadenopathy, fever, pharyngitis, weight loss, and genital lesions (condylomata lata). The rash resolves spontaneously in 2–6 weeks. Neurologic manifestations are rare.
- *Latent syphilis* is usually subclinical, although clinical relapses may occur.
- *Tertiary syphilis* is characterized by slowly progressive signs and symptoms, including gumma formation, cardiovascular disease, and/or CNS changes (neurosyphilis). Such manifestations usually develop 5–20 years after the disease has become latent.

5. *Treponema pallidum* crosses the placenta. Vertical transmission can occur at any time in pregnancy and any stage of the disease, but is most common with primary, secondary or early latent disease (40–50%) compared with late latent or tertiary disease (10%). Fetal infection causes with IUGR, preterm birth, stillbirth, hydrops fetalis, low birthweight, neonatal death, and congenital anomalies. Only 20% of children born to mothers with untreated syphilis will be normal.

6. All pregnant women should have blood taken for serologic screening for syphilis at their first prenatal. Nontreponemal antibody tests should be used for screening, either the Venereal Disease Research Laboratory (VDRL) or rapid plasma reagin (RPR) test. These tests are inexpensive and easy to perform. A positive test should include report of an antibody titer.

7. *Treponema pallidum* cannot be cultured in the laboratory. Confirmation of the diagnosis relies on direct visualization of the organism (by dark-field microscopy or direct fluorescent antibody staining of scrapings or body secretions) or, more commonly, by serologic testing using specific treponemal antibody tests (e.g. fluorescent treponemal antibody absorption (FTA-ABS), microhemagglutination assay for antibodies to *T. pallidum* (MHA-TP) or *T. pallidum* particle agglutination assay (TPPA)). Rarely,

examination of the cerebrospinal fluid may be needed. CSF abnormalities suggestive of infection include an elevated white cell count (>5 cells/μL), elevated total protein (>45 mg/dL), normal glucose concentrations, and a positive CSF VDRL.

8. Treatment of maternal syphilis is critical to prevent congenital infection: 70–100% of infants born to untreated mothers will be infected vs 1–2% of those born to women adequately treated in pregnancy. Note that treatment may precipitate the Jarisch–Herxheimer reaction due to the release of large amounts of treponemal antigen, which, in the latter half of pregnancy, can lead to uterine contractions, preterm labor, and/or nonreassuring fetal testing.

9. *Penicillin is the treatment of choice for syphilis in pregnancy* to treat maternal disease, prevent vertical transmission, and treat established fetal disease. No penicillin-resistant strains of *T. pallidum* have been identified. Second-line agents are not recommended in pregnancy because they are ineffective (erythromycin, clindamycin), contraindicated (tetracycline) or lack sufficient data regarding efficacy (ceftriaxone, azithromycin). The penicillin regimen depends on the stage of disease: (i) benzathine penicillin 2.4 mU intramuscular injection (IMI) × 1 for early disease; (ii) benzathine penicillin 2.4 mU IMI weekly × 3 for latent disease.

10. Approximately 5–10% of pregnant women report an allergy to penicillin. Skin testing to document a true penicillin allergy should be performed in all such women, except those who have had a documented anaphylactic reaction to penicillin. The only satisfactory treatment for penicillin-allergic pregnant patients with syphilis is inpatient desensitization (either oral or subcutaneous) followed by penicillin therapy.

11. Nontreponemal antibody serologic titers (VDRL, RPR) should decrease fourfold by 6 months and become nonreactive by 12–24 months after treatment. Titers that show a fourfold rise or do not decrease appropriately suggest either treatment failure or reinfection. Such women should be treated again, their partners should be treated, and consideration should be given to performing a lumbar puncture to evaluate for CNS involvement.

30 Tuberculosis[1]

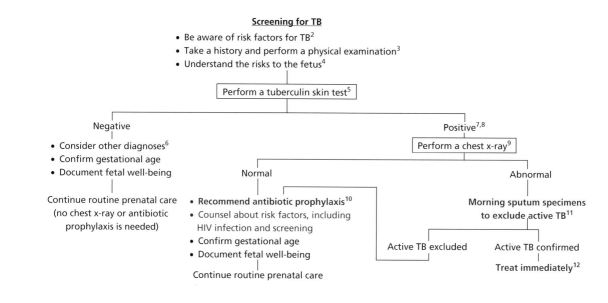

Screening for TB

- Be aware of risk factors for TB[2]
- Take a history and perform a physical examination[3]
- Understand the risks to the fetus[4]

Perform a tuberculin skin test[5]

Negative
- Consider other diagnoses[6]
- Confirm gestational age
- Document fetal well-being

Continue routine prenatal care (no chest x-ray or antibiotic prophylaxis is needed)

Positive[7,8]

Perform a chest x-ray[9]

Normal
- **Recommend antibiotic prophylaxis[10]**
- Counsel about risk factors, including HIV infection and screening
- Confirm gestational age
- Document fetal well-being

Continue routine prenatal care

Abnormal

Morning sputum specimens to exclude active TB[11]

Active TB excluded

Active TB confirmed

Treat immediately[12]

---

1. Tuberculosis (TB) refers to infection with the organism *Myobacterium tuberculosis*. Most cases of TB in immunocompetent adults involve the lungs, but it can affect any organ system. Although it is now rare in developed countries, TB remains one of the leading causes of morbidity and mortality worldwide.

2. Risk factors for TB include: (i) a prior history of TB; (ii) a history of a positive tuberculin skin test; (iii) new immigrants from countries with a high prevalence of TB; (iv) travel to a high-prevalence area; (v) HIV infection; and (vi) a history of homelessness or incarceration. Pregnancy itself does not predispose to infection with TB, although it may be associated with a higher rate of reactivation in women previously infected with TB.

3. A history should include questions about risk factors for TB (above). Symptoms may be nonspecific, including fever, weight loss, malaise, and sweats (especially drenching "night sweats"). In pulmonary TB, additional symptoms may include cough, hemoptysis (coughing blood), and shortness of breath. In extrapulmonary TB, symptoms may include local swelling or pain, a chronically draining lesion, headache or confusion. Most infected women are symptomatic. Physical findings may include focal rales on pulmonary examination, evidence of pleural effusion or a focal mass or lymphadenopathy.

4. Congenital disease resulting from transplacental transmission of TB is rare and occurs almost exclusively when the placenta is actively infected, which is seen more commonly with maternal extrapulmonary disease. As such, pulmonary TB alone poses little risk to the fetus. The greatest risk in women with pulmonary TB is transmission to the infant shortly after birth. Thus, the potential infectiousness of the mother should be resolved prior to delivery.

Obstetric Clinical Algorithms: Management and Evidence. By © E.R. Norwitz, M. Belfort, G.R. Saade and H. Miller.
Published 2010 Blackwell Publishing.

5. All pregnant women should be screened for exposure to TB. Exceptions include: (i) low-risk women who have already had such testing within the preceding year, and (ii) asymptomatic women who have previously had a positive tuberculin test and who have completed a full course of antibiotic prophylaxis. Pregnancy itself does not alter the response to the tuberculin skin test. Such testing involves intradermal (not subcutaneous) injection of purified protein derivative (PPD) and measurement of the extent of induration (skin thickening, not redness) at the injection site 72 hours later.

6. If the patient has pulmonary symptoms, consider other diagnoses such as pneumonia, asthma, and pulmonary embolism.

7. Interpretation of the PPD test depends on the risk status of the patient: (i) in very high-risk women (HIV positive, abnormal chest x-ray, recent contact with an active case of TB), use ≥5 mm induration as positive; (ii) in high-risk women (foreign born, iv drug use, medical conditions or immunosuppressant medications increasing the risk of TB), use ≥10 mm induration as positive; (iii) in low-risk women (no risk factors), use ≥15 mm induration as positive. A positive PPD test implies that a woman has been exposed to *M. tuberculosis*, it does not mean that she has TB *infection*.

8. Bacille Calmette–Guerin (BCG) vaccination is commonly used in developing countries. It does not prevent pulmonary TB, but does prevent complications such as TB meningitis. To maintain its efficacy, BCG should be boosted every 5 years. If >5 years have passed, a positive PPD cannot be attributed to BCG.

9. Chest x-ray is not a good screening tool for TB infection in low-risk populations, but is useful in PPD-positive and symptomatic patients. A normal chest x-ray is reassuring but an abnormal x-ray cannot accurately distinguish between old and active disease. Women may be reluctant to have a chest x-ray in pregnancy. While it does expose the fetus to ionizing radiation, the amount is so small (<1 mRad) as to be nonsignificant. ACOG has stated that up to 5 Rad (5,000 mRad) is completely safe in pregnancy. Waiting until after 12 weeks' gestation and appropriate shielding of the abdomen are reasonable recommendations. If a woman declines a chest x-ray in pregnancy, she should be separated from her baby immediately after birth until active TB infection can be excluded.

10. Women who are PPD positive with a normal chest x-ray require antibiotic prophylaxis. The recommended regimen is isoniazid (INH) 300 mg/day with pyridoxine (to decrease the incidence of INH neurotoxicity) for 9 months. Prophylaxis can be deferred in women over the age of 35. Although INH crosses the placenta, there is no increased toxicity to the fetus. As such, INH can be started in pregnancy. Indeed, if the patient is very high risk (see above), INH should be started immediately. Alternatively, it can be deferred until 6 weeks postpartum; it is not recommended to start INH prophylaxis in the immediate postpartum period because of the increased risk of hepatic toxicity. Breastfeeding is not contraindicated.

11. An abnormal chest x-ray cannot accurately distinguish between old infection (scarring) and active disease. As such, active pulmonary TB disease must be excluded in all asymptomatic patients who are PPD positive with an abnormal chest x-ray. This is done by sputum examination for *M. tuberculosis*. Three negative early morning sputum specimens effectively exclude the diagnosis of active disease. While the sputum is being evaluated, patients should be started on treatment with INH and ethambutol and, if in hospital, should be maintained on contact precautions and in a laminar flow room.

12. If sputum examination confirms active TB, the benefits of treatment in pregnancy dramatically outweigh any potential drug toxicity. Pregnancy does not affect the response to medications, but standard regimens should be modified (e.g. streptomycin is not used because of possible ototoxicity in the fetus). Pregnant women should be treated with a combination of INH, rifampin, and ethambutol for 9 months. Pyrazinamide should be added if drug-resistant TB is suspected.

31 Chorioamnionitis (Intra-amniotic Infection)[1]

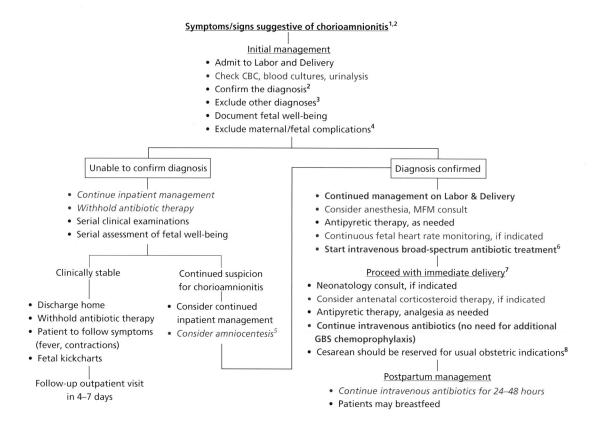

Symptoms/signs suggestive of chorioamnionitis[1,2]

Initial management
- Admit to Labor and Delivery
- Check CBC, blood cultures, urinalysis
- Confirm the diagnosis[2]
- Exclude other diagnoses[3]
- Document fetal well-being
- Exclude maternal/fetal complications[4]

Unable to confirm diagnosis

- *Continue inpatient management*
- *Withhold antibiotic therapy*
- Serial clinical examinations
- Serial assessment of fetal well-being

Clinically stable

- Discharge home
- Withhold antibiotic therapy
- Patient to follow symptoms (fever, contractions)
- Fetal kickcharts

Follow-up outpatient visit in 4–7 days

Continued suspicion for chorioamnionitis

- Consider continued inpatient management
- *Consider amniocentesis[5]*

Diagnosis confirmed

- **Continued management on Labor & Delivery**
- Consider anesthesia, MFM consult
- Antipyretic therapy, as needed
- Continuous fetal heart rate monitoring, if indicated
- **Start intravenous broad-spectrum antibiotic treatment[6]**

Proceed with immediate delivery[7]
- Neonatology consult, if indicated
- Consider antenatal corticosteroid therapy, if indicated
- Antipyretic therapy, analgesia as needed
- **Continue intravenous antibiotics (no need for additional GBS chemoprophylaxis)**
- Cesarean should be reserved for usual obstetric indications[8]

Postpartum management
- *Continue intravenous antibiotics for 24–48 hours*
- Patients may breastfeed

Obstetric Clinical Algorithms: Management and Evidence. By © E.R. Norwitz, M. Belfort, G.R. Saade and H. Miller.
Published 2010 Blackwell Publishing.

1. Chorioamnionitis (intra-amniotic infection) is usually an ascending infection by organisms of the lower genital tract. As such, most intra-amniotic infections are polymicrobial, including such organisms as *E. coli*, *Klebsiella*, *Bacteroides*, GBS, *Fusobacterium*, *Clostridium*, and *Peptostreptococcus*. Mild subclinical infections may be associated with *Mycoplasma*, *Ureaplasma*, and *Fusobacterium*. Risk factors for chorioamnionitis include prolonged rupture of the fetal membranes (>24 hours), multiple digital vaginal examinations, and active vaginal infection (such as bacterial vaginosis). In rare instances (such as listeriosis), maternal bacteremia can seed the amniotic space. Chorioamnionitis complicates approximately 1% of all pregnancies.

2. Chorioamnionitis is a <u>clinical</u> diagnosis characterized by two or more of the following features: maternal fever (>104.0°F orally), fetal tachycardia (>160 bpm), maternal tachycardia (>100 bpm), and uterine tenderness (typically fundal tenderness between contractions). Constitutional symptoms (chills, malaise), uterine contractions, a malodorous vaginal discharge, and an elevated white cell count are common findings but are not required for the diagnosis. There is no place for radiologic imaging studies to confirm the diagnosis. Intra-amniotic infection with *Listeria monocytogenes* is unusual in that the mother is often asymptomatic.

3. The differential diagnosis of chorioamnionitis includes labor and other infectious/inflammatory conditions such as appendicitis, urinary tract infection (cystitis, pyelonephritis), and inflammatory bowel disease.

4. Maternal complications include preterm labor and delivery, increased cesarean delivery rate, postpartum endometritis, pulmonary edema, sepsis, adult respiratory distress syndrome (ARDS), and death. Fetal complications include prematurity, fetal/neonatal sepsis, and increased risk of cerebral palsy.

5. Definitive diagnosis requires a positive amniotic fluid culture. Other features of the amniotic fluid that may suggest infection include glucose ≤20 mg/dL, leukocytes, and bacteria on gram stain. Gram stain alone has a sensitivity of only 30–50%.

6. Although chorioamnionitis cannot be managed expectantly with antibiotics, prompt administration of antibiotics will reduce neonatal sepsis, maternal febrile morbidity, and duration of hospitalization. Intravenous ampicillin 2 g q 4–6 h plus gentamicin 1.5 mg/kg q 8 h (after confirmation of normal renal function) are the antibiotics of choice prior to delivery. Clindamycin or metronidazole should be added immediately after clamping of the cord to further cover anaerobic organisms. Antibiotics should be continued through the postpartum period until the patient is 24–48 hours afebrile and asymptomatic. Longer antibiotic therapy may be required if blood cultures are positive.

7. Once the diagnosis of chorioamnionitis has been established, delivery should be effected regardless of gestational age. Ideally, delivery should be achieved within 8–12 hours. Maternal prognosis is good with prompt diagnosis and treatment. Neonatal mortality and morbidity are related primarily to gestational age.

8. Chorioamnionitis is an indication for delivery but is not in and of itself an indication for cesarean delivery. However, pregnancies complicated by chorioamnionitis are more likely to be delivered abdominally, usually due to nonreassuring fetal testing.

SECTION 4
Antenatal Complications

32 Advanced Maternal Age

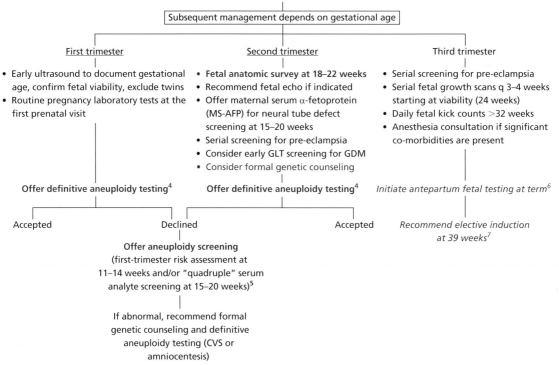

<u>Confirm the diagnosis of advanced maternal age (AMA)[1]</u>

- Take a detailed history and perform a physical examination[2]
- Be aware of the risks of AMA[3]

| Subsequent management depends on gestational age |

First trimester

- Early ultrasound to document gestational age, confirm fetal viability, exclude twins
- Routine pregnancy laboratory tests at the first prenatal visit

Offer definitive aneuploidy testing[4]

Accepted   Declined

Offer aneuploidy screening
(first-trimester risk assessment at 11–14 weeks and/or "quadruple" serum analyte screening at 15–20 weeks)[5]

If abnormal, recommend formal genetic counseling and definitive aneuploidy testing (CVS or amniocentesis)

Second trimester

- **Fetal anatomic survey at 18–22 weeks**
- **Recommend fetal echo if indicated**
- **Offer maternal serum α-fetoprotein (MS-AFP) for neural tube defect screening at 15–20 weeks**
- **Serial screening for pre-eclampsia**
- **Consider early GLT screening for GDM**
- **Consider formal genetic counseling**

Offer definitive aneuploidy testing[4]

Accepted

Third trimester

- Serial screening for pre-eclampsia
- Serial fetal growth scans q 3–4 weeks starting at viability (24 weeks)
- Daily fetal kick counts >32 weeks
- Anesthesia consultation if significant co-morbidities are present

Initiate antepartum fetal testing at term[6]

Recommend elective induction at 39 weeks[7]

Obstetric Clinical Algorithms: Management and Evidence. By © E.R. Norwitz, M. Belfort, G.R. Saade and H. Miller.
Published 2010 Blackwell Publishing.

1. Advanced maternal age (AMA) refers to a woman who is age 35 or older on her estimated date of delivery. Over the last 30 years, there has been a 30% increase in first births among women aged 35–39 years in the US and an even higher increase (70%) among women aged 40–45 years. This change in maternal demographics poses new challenges for prenatal care. It is not clear whether the entity of "advanced paternal age" exists, although there is evidence to suggest that pregnancies fathered by men over 65 years of age are at increased risk of autosomal dominant genetic disorders (such as achondroplasia) and autism.

2. Confirm maternal age. Obtain further details about the timing and mode of conception. For example, if the pregnancy is the result of *in vitro* fertilization with donor oocytes, then the risks of fetal aneuploidy are related to the "age" of the oocytes (i.e. the age of the donor) and not the age of the woman carrying the pregnancy. Physical examination should be focused on identifying underlying co-morbid medical conditions.

3. Advanced maternal age has long been known to be a risk factor for fetal aneuploidy, including trisomy 21 (Down syndrome), trisomy 13, and trisomy 18. In this regard, there is nothing magical about age 35 at delivery. The risk of fetal aneuploidy does not jump up after that date, but increases exponentially with advancing maternal age. The reason why age 35 at delivery was chosen to define AMA is that the risk of identifying a fetal aneuploidy by second-trimester genetic amniocentesis at that maternal age is approximately equal to the procedure-related pregnancy loss rate of amniocentesis (originally estimated at 1 in 270).

In addition to the risk of fetal aneuploidy, AMA is also an independent risk factor for other adverse pregnancy events, including higher rates of spontaneous abortion, spontaneous preterm birth, gestational diabetes mellitus (GDM), gestational hypertension/pre-eclampsia, placenta previa, intrauterine growth restriction (IUGR), and stillbirth/intrauterine fetal death (IUFD). Other maternal complications include an increased risk of cesarean delivery and postpartum hemorrhage. The reason for these increased risks is not clear, although some of these complications can be attributed to the higher incidence of maternal medical disorders with advancing age. The risks of AMA should be reviewed with the couple at their first prenatal visit.

4. In the first trimester, chorionic villous sampling (CVS) can be offered for karyotype analysis at 11–14 weeks gestation. Early amniocentesis (<15 weeks) is associated with increased pregnancy loss and is therefore not recommended. After 15 weeks, ultrasound-guided amniocentesis can be performed and amniocytes isolated for karyotype analysis (see Chapter 50). The procedure-related pregnancy loss rate for both CVA and amniocentesis is estimated at 1 in 400.

5. See Chapter 50.

6. Antenatal fetal testing should be initiated at term (starting at 37–38 weeks gestation). Although there are no clear guidelines, most authorities would recommend weekly nonstress testing (NST) with an assessment of amniotic fluid volume (biophysical profile or Amniotic Fluid Index). If delivery is not achieved by 40 weeks, consider increasing the testing frequency to twice weekly. Immediate delivery is indicated in the setting of nonreassuring fetal testing.

7. Elective induction of labor should be offered to all AMA women at or after 39 weeks gestation with or without cervical ripening. If the patient declines, continued expectant management with fetal testing is appropriate with induction at 40 weeks, but no later than 41 weeks.

33 Antepartum Fetal Testing[1]

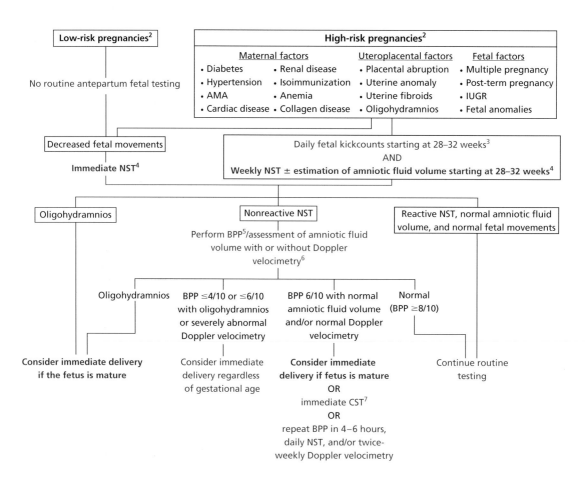

1. Obstetric care providers have two patients: the mother and fetus. Assessment of maternal well-being is relatively easy, but fetal well-being is far more difficult to assess. A number of tests have been developed to confirm fetal well-being prior to the onset of labor. There are many causes of irreversible neonatal cerebral injury, including congenital abnormalities, intracerebral hemorrhage, hypoxic ischemic injury, infection, drugs, trauma, hypotension, and metabolic derangements (such as hypoglycemia and thyroid dysfunction). Antenatal fetal testing cannot predict or reliably detect all of these causes. Moreover, the predictive value of these tests depends on gestational age, the presence or absence of congenital anomalies, and underlying clinical risk factors.

The goal of antepartum fetal surveillance is early identification of a fetus at risk for preventable morbidity or mortality *due specifically to uteroplacental insufficiency*. All antenatal fetal tests make the following assumptions: (i) that pregnancies may be complicated by progressive fetal asphyxia which can lead to fetal death or permanent

Obstetric Clinical Algorithms: Management and Evidence. By © E.R. Norwitz, M. Belfort, G.R. Saade and H. Miller.
Published 2010 Blackwell Publishing.

handicap; (ii) that current antenatal tests can adequately discriminate between asphyxiated and nonasphyxiated fetuses; and (iii) that detection of asphyxia at an early stage can lead to an intervention which is capable of reducing the likelihood of an adverse perinatal outcome. Unfortunately, it is not clear whether any of these assumptions are true. At most, 15% of cerebral palsy is due to birth asphyxia.

2. The designations "low-risk" and "high-risk" pregnancies refer to whether or not pregnancies are at risk of uteroplacental insufficiency.

3. Fetal movement charts ("kickcounts") involve counting the time it takes the fetus to kick 10 times ("count to ten") or counting all fetal movements in 1 hour. Measurements should be repeated twice daily. Use of "kickcounts" in high-risk pregnancies after 28–32 weeks can decrease perinatal mortality fourfold. Although decreased fetal movements may be a sign of fetal compromise, other factors are associated with decreased fetal movements including advancing gestational age, oligohydramnios, smoking, and antenatal corticosteroid therapy.

4. *Non-stress testing* (NST) – also known as cardiotocography (CTG) – refers to changes in the fetal heart rate pattern with time. It reflects maturity of the fetal autonomic nervous system. NST is noninvasive, simple to perform, readily available, and inexpensive. Interpretation is largely subjective. A "reactive" NST (R-NST) – defined as an NST with a normal baseline heart rate (110–160 bpm), moderate variability, and at least two accelerations in 20 min each lasting $\geq$15 s and peaking at $\geq$15 bpm above baseline (or $\geq$10 bpm for $\geq$10 s if <32 weeks) – is reassuring and is associated with normal neurologic outcome. In high-risk pregnancies, weekly NST after 32 weeks has been shown to decrease perinatal mortality. A nonreactive NST (NR-NST) should be interpreted in light of gestational age. Once a R-NST has been documented, it should remain so throughout gestation. A NR-NST at term is associated with poor perinatal outcome in only 20% of cases. Vibroacoustic

stimulation (VAS) refers to the response of the fetal heart rate to a vibroacoustic stimulus. An acceleration on NST ($\geq$15 bpm for $\geq$15 s) is a positive result. It is a useful adjunct to decrease the time to achieve a R-NST and to decrease the proportion of NR-NST at term, thereby precluding the need for further testing.

5. *Biophysical profile* (BPP) refers to a sonographic scoring system designed to assess fetal well-being. The five variables described in the original BPP are: NST, fetal movement, fetal tone, amniotic fluid volume, and fetal breathing. Two points are awarded if the variable is present or normal; 0 points if absent or abnormal. Amniotic fluid volume is the most important variable. More recently, BPP is interpreted without the NST.

6. Umbilical artery *Doppler velocimetry* measurements reflect resistance to blood flow from the fetus to the placenta. Absent or reversed end-diastolic flow (so-called severely abnormal Doppler velocimetry) is associated with poor perinatal outcome in the setting of IUGR, and urgent delivery should be considered regardless of gestational age. It is unclear how to interpret these data in the setting of a normally grown fetus. Abnormal flow in the fetal middle cerebral artery (MCA) and/or ductus venosus may help in the timing of delivery of IUGR fetuses.

7. *Contraction stress test* (CST) – also known as the oxytocin challenge test (OCT) – refers to the response of the fetal heart rate to artificially induced uterine contractions. A minimum of three uterine contractions in 10 min is required to interpret the test. A negative CST (i.e. no decelerations with contractions) is reassuring. A positive CST (i.e. repetitive late or severe variable decelerations with $\geq$50% of contractions) is associated with adverse perinatal outcome in 35–40% of cases. Although the false-positive rate exceeds 50%, a positive CST should result in immediate and urgent delivery. An equivocal CST should be repeated in 24–72 hours. Because this test is time consuming, requires skilled nursing care, and may precipitate "fetal distress" requiring emergent cesarean delivery, it is rarely used in clinical practice.

34 Breast Lesions

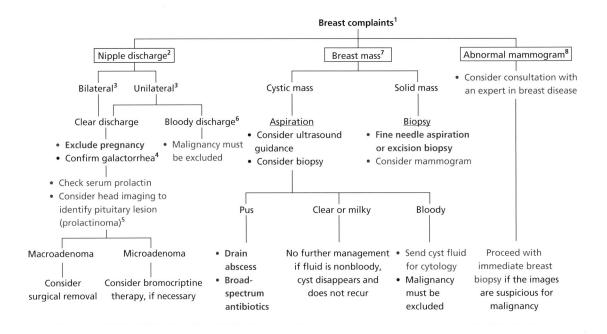

1. A wide range of disorders can present with symptoms relating to the breast, including developmental disorders and diseases of infectious, endocrine, and neoplastic etiology. The presenting symptoms fall into four main categories: nipple discharge, pruritus, pain, and breast masses. Careful attention to history and physical exam as well as selective use of laboratory and imaging studies will allow definitive diagnosis. While the majority of breast conditions are benign, an underlying malignancy should always be excluded. Breast discomfort (mastalgia) may be cyclic or noncyclic. Cyclic mastalgia (breast pain that varies with the menstrual cycle) is not related to cancer, but may be severe enough to require symptomatic treatment. Noncyclic mastalgia should be evaluated further to exclude mastitis, abscess, fat necrosis or trauma. Persistent severe localized breast pain warrants serial clinical breast exams and interval mammograms with or without guided biopsy to exclude malignancy.

2. A detailed history should be taken regarding the character, timing, color, and consistency of the discharge. Spontaneous discharge more likely represents an intraductal growth, whereas discharge only upon stimulation or squeezing of the nipple is less concerning. A thorough clinical breast exam should be performed.

3. Bilateral nipple discharge almost always represents benign disease. Nonmilky, nonbloody bilateral nipple discharge is symptomatic of duct ectasia (plasma cell mastitis) in most cases. Unilateral nipple discharge raises concern

Obstetric Clinical Algorithms: Management and Evidence. By © E.R. Norwitz, M. Belfort, G.R. Saade and H. Miller.
Published 2010 Blackwell Publishing.

about malignancy, but may represent a benign condition (such as intraductal papilloma). Pathologic examination of biopsy material is required to distinguish between these possibilities.

4. Galactorrhea refers to inappropriate production of milk by the breast. It typically presents as a painless, milky discharge from the breasts bilaterally. Microscopic examination of the discharge will stain positive for fat droplets. It may occur during pregnancy or may represent an underlying endocrine disorder. Women with galactorrhea typically have elevated serum prolactin levels, the causes of which include prolactinoma, underlying medical conditions (hypothyroidism, renal failure, encephalitis, meningitis, craniopharyngioma, hypothalamic tumors, hydrocephalus), medications (oral contraceptives, anabolic steroids, medroxyprogesterone acetate, reserpine, omeprazole, calcium channel blockers, opiates, antiemetics, phenothiazines, tricyclic antidepressants, butyrophenones), and other substances (marijuana, alcohol). If pituitary macroadenoma is excluded, the patient has normal menstrual cycles, and the galactorrhea is not socially embarrassing, no treatment is necessary. Bromocriptine can be given if treatment is warranted, and symptoms should resolve within 6–10 weeks. Fewer than 10% of patients will require long-term bromocriptine therapy.

5. Prolactinoma is a prolactin-secreting adenoma of the pituitary gland. Bromocriptine therapy is usually adequate to control symptoms and cause tumor regression. Transsphenoidal resection of the adenoma should be reserved for patients who have macroadenomas (>1.0 cm), have failed medical treatment or have symptoms of headache or evidence of visual field defects (bitemporal hemianopia).

6. A bloody nipple discharge is concerning for cancer. While only 4% of spontaneous, unilateral, bloody discharge represents cancer, a history of a bloody nipple discharge (whether unilateral or bilateral) should be thoroughly evaluated to exclude malignancy. Any elicited discharge should be examined for the presence of blood (by guiac testing) and, if present, should be sent for cytologic examination. If no mass is palpable, imaging studies following injection of dye into the ductal system may outline intraductal irregularities, thereby identifying areas for biopsy.

7. While not all breast masses are cancer, it should be remembered that a palpable mass is the most common presenting symptom of breast cancer. Therefore, reports of a suspected breast mass should always be taken seriously. A detailed history should be taken regarding the timing, character, and consistency of the mass. Associated clinical features may include nipple discharge and pain. The patient's age, parity, menopausal status, personal or family history of cancer, and medication history should also be recorded. The presence of constitutional symptoms (weight loss, anorexia) should be evaluated, since these may point to an underlying malignancy. A detailed clinical breast exam may confirm the presence of the mass as well as its location, size, mobility, consistency, and nodularity. The overlying skin and axillary and supraclavicular lymph nodes should also be examined. Aspiration, imaging (mammography, ultrasound), and biopsy may be necessary to determine what the mass represents.

8. Routine use of screening mammography has led to the increased detection of subclinical abnormalities (such as clustered microcalcifications or asymmetric densities) and an increase in the number of breast biopsies performed. While only approximately 30% of all biopsies of mammographically abnormal lesions are ultimately found to be malignant, mammography may have an important role in detecting early breast cancer. Indeed, 35–50% of early breast cancers are detectable only by mammography. Biopsy of the abnormality may be indicated if the diagnostic mammogram remains suspicious. A negative mammogram does not exclude cancer, since upwards of 40% of breast cancers are detectable only by palpation. Screening mammogram is not routinely indicated in young women (<28 years) or in pregnancy, because of the density of the breast tissue.

35 Cervical Insufficiency

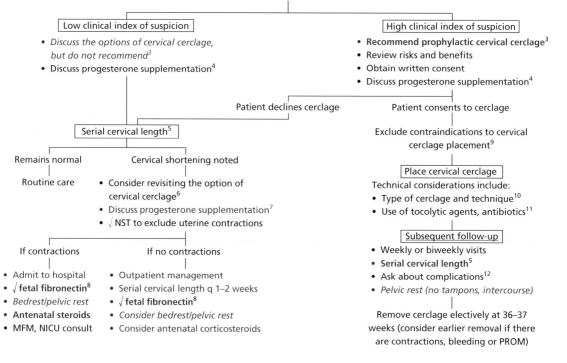

Suspect the diagnosis[1]
- History of prior unexplained mid-trimester pregnancy loss
- Presence or absence of risk factors[2]
- Confirm gestational age
- Document fetal well-being

Low clinical index of suspicion
- *Discuss the options of cervical cerclage, but do not recommend[3]*
- Discuss progesterone supplementation[4]

High clinical index of suspicion
- **Recommend prophylactic cervical cerclage[3]**
- Review risks and benefits
- Obtain written consent
- Discuss progesterone supplementation[4]

Patient declines cerclage

Patient consents to cerclage

Serial cervical length[5]

Remains normal — Routine care

Cervical shortening noted
- Consider revisiting the option of cervical cerclage[6]
- Discuss progesterone supplementation[7]
- √ NST to exclude uterine contractions

Exclude contraindications to cervical cerclage placement[9]

Place cervical cerclage
Technical considerations include:
- Type of cerclage and technique[10]
- Use of tocolytic agents, antibiotics[11]

Subsequent follow-up
- Weekly or biweekly visits
- **Serial cervical length[5]**
- Ask about complications[12]
- *Pelvic rest (no tampons, intercourse)*

Remove cerclage electively at 36–37 weeks (consider earlier removal if there are contractions, bleeding or PROM)

If contractions
- Admit to hospital
- **√ fetal fibronectin[8]**
- *Bedrest/pelvic rest*
- **Antenatal steroids**
- MFM, NICU consult

If no contractions
- Outpatient management
- Serial cervical length q 1–2 weeks
- **√ fetal fibronectin[8]**
- *Consider bedrest/pelvic rest*
- Consider antenatal corticosteroids

---

1. Cervical insufficiency (CI – also known as cervical incompetence) refers to a <u>functional</u> weakness of the cervix resulting in a failure to carry a pregnancy to term. CI is a <u>clinical</u> diagnosis characterized by acute, painless dilation of the cervix usually in the second trimester (16–24 weeks) culminating in membrane prolapse and/or PROM with resultant preterm and often previable delivery. Symptoms may include watery discharge, pelvic pressure, vaginal bleeding or PROM, but most women are asymptomatic.

Uterine contractions are typically absent or minimal. The cause is not known. There is no test in the nonpregnant state that can confirm the diagnosis. CI complicates 0.1–2% of all pregnancies, and is responsible for 15% of births between 16 and 28 weeks' gestation.

2. Risk factors for CI include a prior history of CI, *in utero* diethylstilbestrol (DES) exposure, connective tissue disorders (Ehlers–Danlos syndrome), cervical

---

Obstetric Clinical Algorithms: Management and Evidence. By © E.R. Norwitz, M. Belfort, G.R. Saade and H. Miller.
Published 2010 Blackwell Publishing.

hypoplasia, prior cervical surgery (cone biopsy, loop electrosurgical excision procedure (LEEP)), and (possibly) ≥ 2 late D&E procedures. Most patients with CI have no identifiable risk factors.

3. Prophylactic (elective) cerclage placement at 13–16 weeks is the appropriate treatment for CI, because of the 15–30% risk of recurrence. If the prior preterm birth was due to preterm labor and not CI, then cerclage is not indicated. Cerclage has only been proven effective in women with ≥ 2 mid-trimester pregnancy losses due to CI. Prophylactic cerclage is not indicated for multiple pregnancies or a history of *in utero* DES exposure in the absence of a prior pregnancy loss.

4. Progesterone supplementation (17α-hydroxyprogesterone caproate 250 mg im weekly from 16–20 weeks through 34–36 weeks) can prevent preterm birth in some women at high risk by virtue of a prior unexplained preterm birth. This option should be discussed and the discussion documented.

5. Cervical length (CL) should be measured serially in women at high risk for preterm birth, including a baseline measurement at 16–18 weeks and q 1–3 weeks thereafter depending on the clinical setting. Measurements can be discontinued at 30–32 weeks. Mean CL at 22–24 weeks is 3.5 cm (10th–90th percentile is 2.5–4.5 cm). CL of <2.5 cm is abnormal. CL of <1.5 cm occurs in <2% of women, but is associated with a 60% and 90% risk of preterm birth at <28 weeks and <32 weeks, respectively.

6. Cervical cerclage placement for either asymptomatic cervical shortening (salvage/rescue cerclage) or premature effacement and/or dilation of the cervix (emergent cerclage) is controversial. The weight of evidence in the literature suggests that there is no benefit from such procedures.

7. One study from the UK has suggested that progesterone supplementation (micronized progesterone 200 mg per vaginam daily from 24 weeks through 34 weeks) can prevent preterm birth in some women at high risk by virtue of a short cervix (<1.5 cm) measured on transvaginal ultrasound in the second trimester.

8. See Chapter 52.

9. Absolute contraindications to cerclage include uterine contractions/preterm labor, intra-amniotic/vaginal infection, ruptured membranes, IUFD, major fetal structural/chromosomal anomaly incompatible with life, absence of patient consent, and ≥ 28 weeks' gestation. Relative contraindications include unexplained vaginal bleeding, IUGR, advanced cervical dilation with prolapsing membranes (because of 50% risk of rupture of membranes), and ≥ 24 weeks' gestation.

10. Written consent is required. An ultrasound should be performed prior to placement to confirm fetal viability and exclude major structural anomalies. Regional anesthesia is preferred. A postoperative ultrasound is recommended to confirm fetal well-being. The decision of which nonabsorbable suture and transvaginal cerclage technique to use (Shirodkar, McDonald) is best left to the discretion of the care provider. Shirodkar cerclage is a single suture placed around the cervix at the level of the internal os after surgically reflecting the bladder anteriorly and rectum posteriorly. McDonald cerclage is one or more purse-string sutures around the cervix placed without dissection of the bladder or rectum. These two types of cerclages are likely equally effective. Transabdominal cerclage is a more invasive procedure requiring a laparotomy for placement and subsequent cesarean delivery, and should therefore be reserved for women in whom a transvaginal cerclage is technically impossible to place or who have failed previous transvaginal cerclages.

11. There are insufficient data to recommend routine use of prophylactic antibiotics or tocolytic medications for elective cerclage placement, although there may be some benefit for emergency cerclage.

12. Short-term complications (<24 hours) include excessive blood loss, PROM, and pregnancy loss (3–20%). Long-term complications include cervical lacerations (3–4%), chorioamnionitis (4%), cervical stenosis (1%), and bladder pain and migration of the suture (rare). Puerperal infection is twice as common in women with a cerclage (6%).

36 First-trimester Vaginal Bleeding

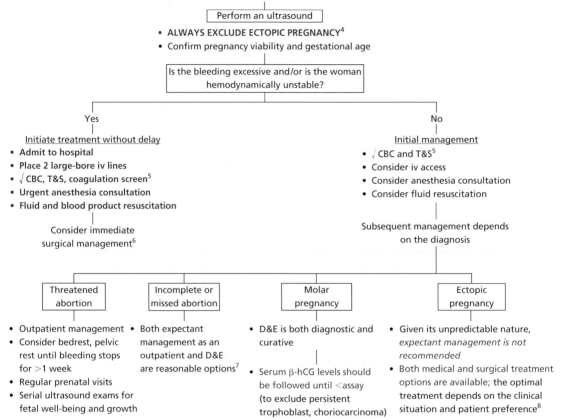

Reported first-trimester vaginal bleeding

- Confirm pregnancy[1]
- Take a detailed history and perform a physical examination[2]
- Consider differential diagnosis of first-trimester vaginal bleeding[3]

Perform an ultrasound

- **ALWAYS EXCLUDE ECTOPIC PREGNANCY[4]**
- Confirm pregnancy viability and gestational age

Is the bleeding excessive and/or is the woman hemodynamically unstable?

Yes

Initiate treatment without delay
- Admit to hospital
- Place 2 large-bore iv lines
- √ CBC, T&S, coagulation screen[5]
- Urgent anesthesia consultation
- Fluid and blood product resuscitation

Consider immediate surgical management[6]

No

Initial management
- √ CBC and T&S[5]
- Consider iv access
- Consider anesthesia consultation
- Consider fluid resuscitation

Subsequent management depends on the diagnosis

| Threatened abortion | Incomplete or missed abortion | Molar pregnancy | Ectopic pregnancy |

Threatened abortion
- Outpatient management
- Consider bedrest, pelvic rest until bleeding stops for >1 week
- Regular prenatal visits
- Serial ultrasound exams for fetal well-being and growth

Incomplete or missed abortion
- Both expectant management as an outpatient and D&E are reasonable options[7]

Molar pregnancy
- D&E is both diagnostic and curative
- Serum β-hCG levels should be followed until <assay (to exclude persistent trophoblast, choriocarcinoma)

Ectopic pregnancy
- Given its unpredictable nature, *expectant management is not recommended*
- Both medical and surgical treatment options are available; the optimal treatment depends on the clinical situation and patient preference[8]

1. A positive serum β-hCG (>5 mIU/mL) confirms the presence of trophoblast tissue (although, in the case of complete abortion, the tissue may already have been passed). High levels of β-hCG suggest a molar pregnancy. Very rarely, β-hCG may be a marker of an ovarian tumor.

2. Bleeding in the first trimester is common; 15–20% of clinically diagnosed pregnancies end in miscarriage. The timing, extent, and severity of the bleeding should

be documented. Maternal vital signs should be taken to rule out hemodynamic instability. Speculum examination allows visualization of the cervix and potentially the location of products of conception. Bimanual exam may help estimate gestational age and identify an adnexal masses or tenderness.

3. The differential diagnosis of first-trimester vaginal bleeding includes: (i) a threatened abortion (defined as a viable

Obstetric Clinical Algorithms: Management and Evidence. By © E.R. Norwitz, M. Belfort, G.R. Saade and H. Miller.
Published 2010 Blackwell Publishing.

intrauterine pregnancy <20 weeks with a closed cervix), incomplete abortion (viable intrauterine pregnancy with an open cervix), missed abortion (nonviable intrauterine pregnancy) or complete abortion (complete passage of an intrauterine pregnancy and closure of the cervix); (ii) ectopic pregnancy (implantation of the pregnancy outside the uterine cavity, including fallopian tubes, cornua, cervix or ovary); (iii) gestational trophoblastic disease (molar pregnancy); and (iv) less commonly, an "implantation bleed," a cervical or vaginal lesion (such as a cervical erosion or postcoital bleeding), and rectal bleeding (hemorrhoids).

4. All first-trimester vaginal bleeding should be regarded as an *ectopic pregnancy* until proven otherwise. Failure to promptly diagnose and manage an ectopic pregnancy can be catastrophic. Ectopic pregnancy accounts for 10% of all pregnancy-related maternal deaths, and is the most common cause of maternal death in the first half of pregnancy. Abdominal pain, absence of menses, and irregular vaginal bleeding (usually spotting) are the main symptoms. The most common presenting sign in a woman with symptomatic ectopic pregnancy is abdominal tenderness, and 50% will have a palpable adnexal mass. Ruptured ectopic pregnancies cause shoulder pain in 10–20% of cases as a result of diaphragmatic irritation from the hemoperitoneum. Profound intraperitoneal hemorrhage can lead to tachycardia and hypotension. The amount of vaginal bleeding is not a reliable indicator of the severity of the hemorrhage since bleeding is often concealed. The primary goal of ultrasound is to confirm an intrauterine pregnancy, which should be evident by transabdominal ultrasound at a serum β-hCG level of $\geq$6000 mIU/mL and by transvaginal ultrasound at a serum β-hCG level of $\geq$1200 mIU/mL (approximately 5 weeks from LMP). The absence of an intrauterine pregnancy on ultrasound with a positive serum β-hCG level should raise the suspicion of an ectopic pregnancy. Only rarely will the ectopic pregnancy itself be visible on ultrasound. The presence of free fluid (blood) in the abdomen suggests a ruptured ectopic or ruptured ovarian cyst.

5. If the patient is Rh negative, she should receive anti-Rh[D]-immunoglobulin (RhoGAM) 300 µg IM to prevent Rh isoimmunization.

6. The nature of the surgical procedure will depend on the diagnosis: (i) D&E if an incomplete abortion is suspected and (ii) laparoscopy and/or explorative laparotomy if a ruptured ectopic pregnancy or ovarian cyst is diagnosed.

7. If the patient is hemodynamically stable with minimal bleeding, expectant management on an outpatient basis is reasonable and will likely avoid a surgical procedure. Only 10% of such women will subsequently require a D&E for excessive vaginal bleeding.

8. Goals of management for an ectopic pregnancy are to prevent maternal mortality, reduce morbidity, and preserve fertility. Once the diagnosis is confirmed, expectant management is rarely justified. Most (95%) ectopic pregnancies occur in the fallopian tubes. Treatment options for such pregnancies include the following.

- *Methotrexate (MTX)* (50 mg/m^2 im) is an effective treatment for patients who are hemodynamically stable without evidence of rupture, compliant, and who meet selection criteria (below). The dose is administered on day 1, but serum β-hCG levels typically continue to rise for several days thereafter. An acceptable response is defined as a $\geq$15% decrease in serum β-hCG levels from day 4 to day 7. β-hCG levels should thereafter be followed weekly. Most cases will be successfully treated with one dose of MTX, but up to 25% will require two or more doses if the serial β-hCG levels plateau or rise. Patients with a gestational sac >3.5 cm, starting β-hCG > 6000 mIU/mL or fetal cardiac motion evident on ultrasound are at higher risk for MTX failure and should be considered for surgical management. Side-effects of MTX are generally mild and include nausea, vomiting, bloating, and transient transaminitis. Increased abdominal pain will occur in up to 75% of patients due to tubal abortion and serosal irritation or distension of the fallopian tube. All MTX patients should be closely monitored due to the risk of rupture and hemorrhage.
- *Surgical therapy.* Definitive surgery (salpingectomy) is the treatment of choice for women who are not hemodynamically stable. Conservative surgery is appropriate for the hemodynamically stable patient. Laparoscopic salpingostomy and removal of the products of conception is the most common procedure. The injection of vasopressin prior to the linear incision can be used to decrease bleeding. Serum β-hCG levels must be followed until undetectable in conservatively managed patients because 5–10% will develop a persistent ectopic pregnancy which may require further treatment with MTX. Failure to achieve hemostasis is the only indication for oophorectomy.

37 Higher-order Multiple Pregnancy

Suspected high-order multiple pregnancy[1]

- Take a detailed history and perform a physical examination[2]
- Be aware of risk factors for multiple pregnancy[3]

Perform an ultrasound[4]

Diagnosis not confirmed

- Exclude other causes of excessive uterine size (e.g. wrong dates, fibroids, polyhydramnios)
- Confirm fetal well-being
- Document gestational age
- Repeat ultrasound examinations as clinically indicated

Continue routine prenatal care

Diagnosis confirmed

Initial management

- Confirm fetal well-being
- Document gestational age
- Consider neonatology, MFM, and anesthesia consults if indicated
- **Determine zygosity and chorionicity**

Subsequent evaluation

- Review risks of higher-order multiple pregnancy[5]
- Screen for fetal structural anomalies[6]
- Screen for fetal aneuploidy[7]

Offer/recommend multifetal pregnancy reduction[8]

Multifetal pregnancy reduction to twins

- **Consider serial cervical length ± fetal fibronectin (fFN)**
- Serial growth scans every 3–4 weeks starting in second trimester
- Consider weekly fetal testing >34 weeks

Intrapartum considerations

- Consider elective delivery at or after 38 weeks (no amniocentesis for fetal lung maturity (FLM))
- Document fetal presentation and EFW
- Consider continuous intrapartum fetal monitoring

Review mode of delivery[9]

Declined

- **Serial cervical length ± fFN**
- Serial growth scans every 2 weeks starting in second trimester
- Consider weekly fetal testing >28 weeks

- *Follow closely for evidence of preterm labor and other maternal complications*
- Consider empiric antepartum corticosteroids and follow-up neonatology consultation
- Document serial fetal presentation and EFW

Deliver by cesarean[9]

Obstetric Clinical Algorithms: Management and Evidence. By © E.R. Norwitz, M. Belfort, G.R. Saade and H. Miller.
Published 2010 Blackwell Publishing.

1. Multiple pregnancies complicate 1–2% of all deliveries and are becoming increasingly common, primarily as a result of assisted reproductive technology (ART). This is especially true of higher-order multiple pregnancies (triplets and up) which now constitute 0.1–0.3% of all births.

2. Multiple pregnancy should be suspected in women with excessive symptoms of pregnancy (e.g. nausea and vomiting) or uterine size larger than expected for gestational age.

3. Risk factors for multiple pregnancy include a family or personal history of multiple pregnancy (except monozygous twins), advanced maternal age, multiparity, African-American race, and ART. The vast majority of higher-order multiple pregnancies result from ART. In this regard, ovulation induction/intrauterine insemination poses a higher risk than *in vitro* fertilization (IVF).

4. Ultrasound will confirm the diagnosis, gestational age, and fetal well-being, and determine the chorionicity (arrangement of membranes in multiple pregnancies).

5. Antepartum complications develop in 80% of multiple pregnancies versus 20–30% of singleton gestations. Preterm delivery is the most common complication, and the risk of preterm delivery increases as fetal number increases: the average length of gestation is 40 weeks in singletons, 37 weeks in twins, 33 weeks in triplets, and 29 weeks in quadruplets. Fetal growth discordance (defined as $\geq$25% difference in EFW) is associated with a significant increase in perinatal mortality. Maternal complications include an increased risk of gestational diabetes, pre-eclampsia, preterm premature rupture of membranes, anemia, cholestasis of pregnancy, cesarean delivery (due primarily to malpresentation), and postpartum hemorrhage. Other fetal complications include an increased risk of fetal structural anomalies, IUFD of one or both twins (see Chapter 39), twin-to-twin transfusion syndrome (TTTS), twin reversed arterial perfusion (TRAP) sequence, and cord entanglement (see Chapter 57).

6. Multiple pregnancies are at increased risk of fetal structural anomalies compared with singletons. A detailed fetal anatomic survey of each fetus is indicated at 18–20 weeks.

Fetal echocardiography is not routinely recommended in multiple pregnancies, but is indicated if the conception was by IVF.

7. Maternal serum α-fetoprotein (MS-AFP), "quadruple panel" serum analyte screening (MS-AFP, estriol, hCG, and inhibin A), and first-trimester risk assessment (nuchal translucency (NT) + serum PAPP-A and β-hCG) have not been adequately validated in higher-order multiple pregnancies. As such, NT alone has become the preferred aneuploidy screening test for higher-order multiple pregnancies. CVS and amniocentesis can be offered for definitive karyotype analysis, but are associated with a procedure-related pregnancy loss rate estimated at 1 in 400.

8. Ten to 15% of higher-order multiple pregnancies will reduce spontaneously during the first trimester. If not, the option of multifetal pregnancy reduction (MFPR) to twins at 13–15 weeks should be offered. The benefits of MFPR include increased length of gestation, increased birthweight, and reduced prematurity and perinatal mortality and mortality. For quadruplet pregnancies and upward, the benefits of MFPR clearly outweigh the risks. In the absence of fetal anomaly, no clear benefit has been demonstrated for reduction of twins to a singleton. Whether triplet pregnancies benefit from MFPR to twins, however, remains controversial. Overall, reduction of triplets to twins seems to result in a more satisfactory pregnancy outcome. The procedure-related pregnancy loss rate prior to 20 weeks may be as high as 15% (range 5–35%), which is comparable to the background spontaneous loss rate for higher-order multiple pregnancies. However, the fetal loss rate increases with advancing gestation at the time of the reduction. MFPR should be distinguished from selective fetal reduction in which one fetus is selectively terminated because of a known structural or chromosomal abnormality.

9. Route of delivery depends on fetal number, gestational age, EFW, presentation, and maternal and fetal well-being (see Chapter 62). Cesarean delivery has traditionally been recommended for all higher-order multiple pregnancies, although vaginal delivery may be appropriate in selected patients.

38 Hyperemesis Gravidarum

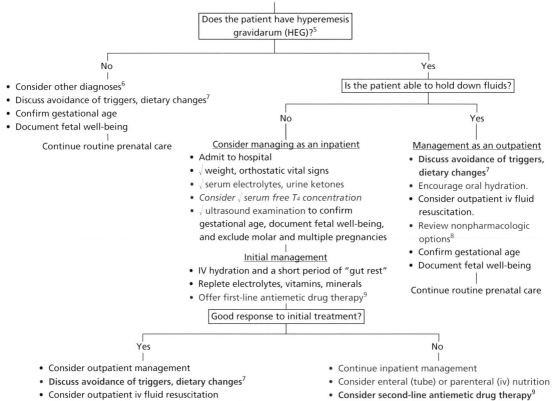

Nausea and vomiting in pregnancy (NVP)

- Understand the pathophysiology of NVP[1]
- Exclude underlying pathologic conditions[2]
- Be aware of risk factors for NVP[3]
- Discuss strategies for prevention[4]

Does the patient have hyperemesis gravidarum (HEG)?[5]

No

- Consider other diagnoses[6]
- Discuss avoidance of triggers, dietary changes[7]
- Confirm gestational age
- Document fetal well-being

Continue routine prenatal care

Yes

Is the patient able to hold down fluids?

No

Consider managing as an inpatient
- Admit to hospital
- √ weight, orthostatic vital signs
- √ serum electrolytes, urine ketones
- *Consider √ serum free T4 concentration*
- √ ultrasound examination to confirm gestational age, document fetal well-being, and exclude molar and multiple pregnancies

Initial management
- IV hydration and a short period of "gut rest"
- Replete electrolytes, vitamins, minerals
- Offer first-line antiemetic drug therapy[9]

Good response to initial treatment?

Yes
- Consider outpatient management
- **Discuss avoidance of triggers, dietary changes[7]**
- Consider outpatient iv fluid resuscitation
- Continue antiemetic drug therapy, as needed[9]

No
- Continue inpatient management
- Consider enteral (tube) or parenteral (iv) nutrition
- **Consider second-line antiemetic drug therapy[9]**
- Pregnancy termination may be a last resort

Yes

Management as an outpatient
- **Discuss avoidance of triggers, dietary changes[7]**
- Encourage oral hydration.
- Consider outpatient iv fluid resuscitation.
- Review nonpharmacologic options[8]
- Confirm gestational age
- Document fetal well-being

Continue routine prenatal care

Obstetric Clinical Algorithms: Management and Evidence. By © E.R. Norwitz, M. Belfort, G.R. Saade and H. Miller.
Published 2010 Blackwell Publishing.

1. Some degree of nausea and vomiting in pregnancy (NVP) or "morning sickness" occurs in >80% of all pregnancies. The mean onset of symptoms is 5–6 weeks, peaking at 9 weeks, and usually abating by 16–18 weeks; however, symptoms continue into the third trimester in 15–20% of women and 5% have symptoms that persist to term. The cause of NVP is not known, although it is thought to be related to hCG production. NVP is not a sign of an unhealthy pregnancy; in fact, pregnancies complicated by NVP have a better outcome than those that are not, with lower rates of miscarriage and stillbirth.

2. Conditions that may present with severe NVP include molar pregnancy, higher-order multiple pregnancy, and women with theca lutein cysts. An ultrasound can exclude these underlying conditions.

3. Risk factors for NVP include: (i) severe NVP in a prior pregnancy (recurrence rate is 15–20%), (ii) nausea and vomiting after estrogen exposure (such as combined oral contraceptive pill), with motion sickness, with migraine or with exposure to certain tastes, (iii) pre-existing psychiatric disorder, (iv) diabetes, and (v) female fetus. A number of protective factors have also been identified, including anosmia (inability to smell), advanced maternal age, and smoking.

4. Several strategies have been tried to prevent NVP, but most have been shown to be no better than placebo. The only intervention that may be somewhat effective in preventing NVP is multivitamin supplementation from the time of conception.

5. Hyperemesis gravidarum (HEG) refers to the severe end of the spectrum of NVP, and complicates 0.3–2% of all pregnancies. It is a clinical diagnosis made in the first trimester and characterized by three criteria: (i) persistent vomiting, (ii) weight loss >5% of pre-pregnancy body weight, and (iii) ketonuria. A number of laboratory abnormalities have been described in the setting of HEG, including electrolyte derangements (hypokalemia, metabolic alkalosis), hemoconcentration (increase in hematocrit), abnormal liver enzyme (elevated ALT and mild hyperbilirubinemia), and hyperthyroidism (mildly elevated free T_4 and depressed TSH, although patients are clinically euthyroid and do not need treatment). However, none of these abnormalities is diagnostic of HEG.

6. The differential diagnosis of HEG is extensive, and includes medication-induced nausea and vomiting, infections (gastroenteritis), small bowel obstruction, peptic ulcer disease, inflammatory bowel disease, and (rarely) central nervous system disorders, malignancies, endocrine/metabolic derangements. After 20 weeks, pre-eclampsia must always be excluded. NVP predating pregnancy or with abdominal pain, fever or neurologic signs suggests an alternative cause.

7. Patients should be counseled about avoidance of environmental triggers for NVP, including odors (coffee, perfume, food, smoke), noise, and visual or physical motion (flickering lights). Dietary changes may relieve NVP in some women, such as frequent, small, high-carbohydrate/low-fat meals; elimination of spicy foods; eating salty or high-protein meals and cold, carbonated, or sour fluids (ginger ale, lemonade). Powdered ginger (1 g daily) and foods containing ginger (ginger lollipops) have been shown to be effective in mild NVP.

8. Nonpharmacologic interventions (such as P6 acupuncture, acupressure wristbands, hypnosis, and psychotherapy) have been proposed to treat mild NVP, but with variable results. Meta-analyses of randomized trials show no significant benefit over sham therapy.

9. Several drugs have been shown to be more effective than placebo in treating NVP with few side-effects and no increased risk of congenital anomalies. A stepwise approach to antiemetic therapy is recommended. *First-line agents* include: (i) pyridoxine (vitamin B6) (10–25 mg q 8 h po) with or without the antihistamine doxylamine succinate (20 mg); (ii) antihistamines (H_1-receptor antagonists) such as promethazine (12.5–25 mg q 4 h po/im/pr). *Second-line agents* include: (i) the selective 5-HT3 serotonin receptor antagonist ondansetron (8 mg q 12 h po/im); (ii) dopamine antagonists such as metoclopramide (5–10 mg q 8 h po/iv), prochlorperazine (5–10 mg q 3–4 h po/im or 25 mg q 12 h pr), phenothiazines or droperidol; and (iii) a short course of corticosteroids (methylprednisolone 16 mg q 8 h po/iv × 3–14 days). The efficacy of corticosteroids is unproven and it has been associated with preterm premature rupture of membranes (PPROM) and oral clefts when administered <10 weeks of gestation; as such, they should be used only as a last resort.

39 Intrauterine Fetal Demise

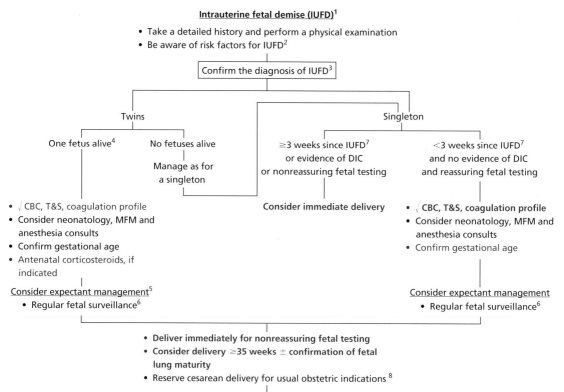

Intrauterine fetal demise (IUFD)[1]
- Take a detailed history and perform a physical examination
- Be aware of risk factors for IUFD[2]

Confirm the diagnosis of IUFD[3]

Twins

One fetus alive[4]

No fetuses alive

Manage as for a singleton

Singleton

≥3 weeks since IUFD[7] or evidence of DIC or nonreassuring fetal testing

<3 weeks since IUFD[7] and no evidence of DIC and reassuring fetal testing

- √ CBC, T&S, coagulation profile
- Consider neonatology, MFM and anesthesia consults
- Confirm gestational age
- Antenatal corticosteroids, if indicated

Consider immediate delivery

- √ CBC, T&S, coagulation profile
- Consider neonatology, MFM and anesthesia consults
- Confirm gestational age

Consider expectant management[5]
- Regular fetal surveillance[6]

Consider expectant management
- Regular fetal surveillance[6]

- **Deliver immediately for nonreassuring fetal testing**
- **Consider delivery ≥35 weeks ± confirmation of fetal lung maturity**
- **Reserve cesarean delivery for usual obstetric indications** [8]

After delivery, attempt to determine the cause of IUFD[9]

Obstetric Clinical Algorithms: Management and Evidence. By © E.R. Norwitz, M. Belfort, G.R. Saade and H. Miller.
Published 2010 Blackwell Publishing.

1. Intrauterine fetal demise (IUFD), also known as stillbirth, is defined in the United States as fetal demise after 20 weeks' gestation and prior to delivery.

2. Risk factors for IUFD include extremes of maternal age, multiple pregnancy, post-term pregnancy, male fetus, fetal macrosomia, and maternal disease such as pregestational diabetes, systemic lupus erythematosus (SLE), and pre-eclampsia.

3. The inability to identify fetal heart tones or the absence of uterine growth may suggest the diagnosis. Ultrasound is the gold standard to confirm an IUFD by documenting the absence of fetal cardiac activity. Other sonographic findings in later pregnancy may include scalp edema, overlapping sutures, and fetal maceration.

4. The death of one twin confers an increased risk of major morbidity to the surviving twin including IUFD, neurologic injury, multiorgan system failure, thrombosis, distal limb necrosis, placental abruption, and premature labor.

5. Prognosis for the surviving twin depends on the cause of death, gestational age, chorionicity, and time interval between death of the first twin and delivery of the second. *Dizygous twin pregnancies* do not share a circulation, and death of one twin may have little impact on the surviving twin. The dead twin may be resorbed completely or become compressed and incorporated into the membranes (*fetus papyraceus*). Disseminated intravascular coagulopathy (DIC) in the surviving fetus and/or mother is rare. On the other hand, some degree of shared circulation can be demonstrated in almost all *monozygous twin pregnancies*, and death of one fetus in this setting carries an increased risk of death of its co-twin due to profound hypotension and/or transfer of thromboplastic proteins from the dead fetus to the live fetus. If it survives, the co-twin has a 40% risk of developing neurologic injury (multicystic encephalomalacia), which may not be prevented by immediate delivery. Therefore, management of a surviving co-twin depends on chorionicity and gestational age.

6. Fetal surveillance should be instituted, including daily kickcharts and weekly or twice-weekly nonstress testing/biophysical profile.

7. Approximately 20–25% of women who retain a dead singleton fetus for longer than 3 weeks will develop DIC due to excessive consumption of clotting factors. Therefore, delivery should be effected within this time period.

8. Every effort should be made to avoid cesarean delivery in the setting of IUFD. As such, expectant management is often recommended. Latency (the period from fetal demise to delivery) varies depending on the underlying cause and gestational age. In general, the earlier the gestational age, the longer the latency period. Overall, >90% of women will go into spontaneous labor within 2 weeks of a singleton fetal death. However, many women find the prospect of carrying a dead fetus distressing and want the pregnancy terminated as soon as possible. Management options include surgical dilation and evacuation or induction of labor with cervical ripening, if indicated.

9. Causes of IUFD can be identified in only around 50% of cases. Pathologic examination of the fetus (autopsy) and placenta/fetal membranes is the single most useful test to identify a cause for the IUFD. Fetal karyotyping should be considered in all cases of fetal death to identify chromosomal abnormalities, particularly in cases with documented fetal structural abnormalities. Approximately 5–10% of stillborn fetuses have an abnormal karyotype. Amniocentesis may be recommended to salvage viable amniocytes for cytogenetic analysis prior to delivery. Trafficking of fetal cells into the maternal circulation occurs in all pregnancies, but is usually minimal (<0.1 mL total volume). In rare instances, fetal-maternal hemorrhage may be massive, leading to fetal demise. The Kleihauer–Betke (acid elution) test or flow cytometric analysis of maternal blood may allow for an estimation of the volume of fetal blood in the maternal circulation, but should ideally be drawn within hours of the suspected bleeding episode due to the rapid clearance of fetal cells from maternal circulation. Intra-amniotic infection resulting in fetal death is usually evident on clinical exam. Placental membrane culture and autopsy examination of the fetus, placenta/fetal membranes, and umbilical cord may be useful. Fetal X-rays or MRI may sometimes be valuable if autopsy is declined. Other conditions that should be considered in the setting of IUFD include pre-eclampsia (especially in the setting of intrauterine growth restriction) and maternal diabetes.

40 Intrauterine Growth Restriction

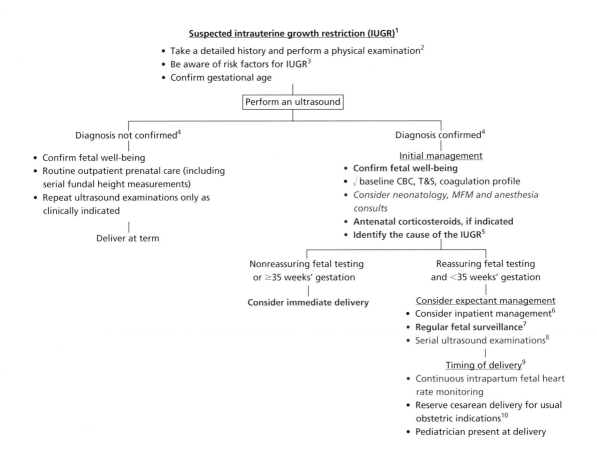

Suspected intrauterine growth restriction (IUGR)[1]
- Take a detailed history and perform a physical examination[2]
- Be aware of risk factors for IUGR[3]
- Confirm gestational age

Perform an ultrasound

Diagnosis not confirmed[4]
- Confirm fetal well-being
- Routine outpatient prenatal care (including serial fundal height measurements)
- Repeat ultrasound examinations only as clinically indicated

Deliver at term

Diagnosis confirmed[4]

Initial management
- **Confirm fetal well-being**
- √ baseline CBC, T&S, coagulation profile
- *Consider neonatology, MFM and anesthesia consults*
- **Antenatal corticosteroids, if indicated**
- **Identify the cause of the IUGR[5]**

Nonreassuring fetal testing or ≥35 weeks' gestation

Consider immediate delivery

Reassuring fetal testing and <35 weeks' gestation

Consider expectant management
- Consider inpatient management[6]
- **Regular fetal surveillance[7]**
- Serial ultrasound examinations[8]

Timing of delivery[9]
- Continuous intrapartum fetal heart rate monitoring
- Reserve cesarean delivery for usual obstetric indications[10]
- Pediatrician present at delivery

1. Intrauterine growth restriction (IUGR) refers to any fetus that fails to reach its full growth potential. In the United States, approximately 4–8% of fetuses are diagnosed with IUGR. IUGR fetuses have higher rates of perinatal morbidity and mortality as compared with appropriate for gestational age (AGA) fetuses for any given gestational age. Neonatal morbidity (meconium aspiration syndrome, hypoglycemia, polycythemia, pulmonary hemorrhage) may be present in up to 50% of IUGR neonates. Premature IUGR infants also have difficulty with nutritional support, and many develop feeding intolerance and failure to thrive in the neonatal intensive care unit. Long-term studies show a twofold increased incidence of cerebral dysfunction (ranging from minor learning disability to cerebral palsy) in IUGR infants delivered at term, and an even higher incidence if the infant was

Obstetric Clinical Algorithms: Management and Evidence. By © E.R. Norwitz, M. Belfort, G.R. Saade and H. Miller.
Published 2010 Blackwell Publishing.

born preterm. Epidemiologic studies also suggest that these infants may be at higher risk for developing chronic disease in adulthood such as diabetes, hypertension, stroke, and coronary heart disease.

2. The clinical diagnosis of IUGR is difficult, and physical examination alone will fail to identify over 50% of IUGR fetuses. If the fundal height measurement is significantly less than expected (<3–4 cm for gestational age), an ultrasound examination should be performed.

3. Risk factors for IUGR include extremes of maternal age, a prior IUGR pregnancy, multiple pregnancy, fetal infection, placental abruption (decidual hemorrhage), inherited thrombophilia (such as factor V Leiden, prothrombin gene mutation), and maternal disease such as pregestational diabetes, SLE, antiphospholipid antibody syndrome, chronic hypertension, unexplained proteinuria, and pre-eclampsia.

4. IUGR is a <u>radiologic</u> diagnosis that requires either (i) an estimated fetal weight (EFW) <3rd percentile (2 standard deviations from the mean) for gestational age, or (ii) an EFW <10th percentile for gestational age along with evidence of fetal compromise such as oligohydramnios or abnormal umbilical artery Doppler velocimetry. As such, accurate gestational age dating is a prerequisite for the diagnosis. A small calcified (Grade 3) placenta and/or a small biparietal circumference (i.e. head circumference/abdominal circumference ratio >95th percentile for gestational age) are other sonographic features suggestive of IUGR, but are not diagnostic. Fetuses who have an EFW between the 3rd and 10th percentiles without evidence of compromise should be referred to as SGA (small for gestational age), and not IUGR.

5. Intrauterine growth restriction likely represents the clinical end-point of many different fetal, uteroplacental, and maternal conditions. Every effort should be made to determine the cause prior to delivery. The most common causes include uteroplacental insufficiency (>50%), genetic factors (5–15%), drug or toxin exposure (5–15%), congenital infection (2–5%), multiple pregnancy (2–3%), malnutrition (2–3%), and fetal structural anomalies (1–2%). As such, investigations should include a detailed fetal anatomic survey including an echocardiogram to exclude a fetal cardiac anomaly, amniocentesis for fetal karyotype (especially if there is a fetal structural anomaly), and maternal serologic testing for TORCH infections (especially if there is fetal liver or cerebral calcification on ultrasound). In addition, pre-eclampsia and antiphospholipid antibody syndrome should be excluded.

6. Inpatient management, bedrest, and medications (such as low-dose aspirin) have not been shown to significantly improve perinatal outcome, but are often recommended. Inpatient management does allow for closer fetal surveillance. IUGR may be the first manifestation of pre-eclampsia, and such pregnancies should be followed on a regular basis to exclude this complication.

7. Fetal surveillance should be instituted immediately, including daily kickcounts and weekly or twice-weekly nonstress testing and/or biophysical profile.

8. Serial growth scans should be performed every 2–3 weeks. More regular ultrasound examinations (at least twice weekly) are indicated to document amniotic fluid volume and/or perform Doppler velocimetry of the umbilical artery, middle cerebral artery (MCA), and ductus venosus.

9. Appropriate timing of delivery is critical to optimizing perinatal outcome in the setting of IUGR, and is dependent in large part on gestational age. Immediate delivery should be considered in the following situations: (i) gestational age ≥35 weeks; (ii) absent interval growth on ultrasound over a 2–3-week period; (iii) pre-existing maternal disease (such as severe pre-eclampsia); (iv) nonreassuring fetal testing (such as a positive contraction stress test (CST), absent variability with repetitive late or variable decelerations); and/or (v) absent or reversed end-diastolic flow on umbilical artery Doppler velocimetry.

10. Intrauterine growth restriction fetuses can undergo vaginal delivery, and cesarean delivery should be reserved for the usual obstetric indications. That said, 50–80% of IUGR fetuses will not tolerate labor and will require delivery by cesarean.

41 Isoimmunization

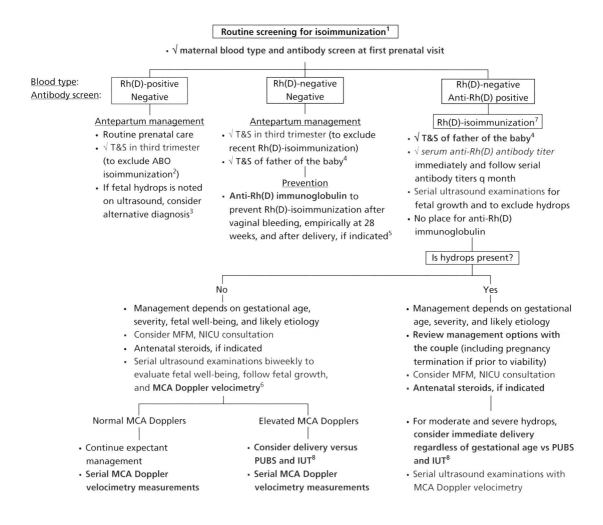

Routine screening for isoimmunization[1]

• √ maternal blood type and antibody screen at first prenatal visit

Blood type: | Rh(D)-positive Negative | Rh(D)-negative Negative | Rh(D)-negative Anti-Rh(D) positive
Antibody screen:

Rh(D)-positive / Negative

Antepartum management
• Routine prenatal care
• √ T&S in third trimester (to exclude ABO isoimmunization[2])
• If fetal hydrops is noted on ultrasound, consider alternative diagnosis[3]

Rh(D)-negative / Negative

Antepartum management
• √ T&S in third trimester (to exclude recent Rh(D)-isoimmunization)
• √ T&S of father of the baby[4]

Prevention
• **Anti-Rh(D) immunoglobulin** to prevent Rh(D)-isoimmunization after vaginal bleeding, empirically at 28 weeks, and after delivery, if indicated[5]

Rh(D)-negative / Anti-Rh(D) positive

Rh(D)-isoimmunization[7]
• √ **T&S of father of the baby[4]**
• √ *serum anti-Rh(D) antibody titer* immediately and follow serial antibody titers q month
• Serial ultrasound examinations for fetal growth and to exclude hydrops
• No place for anti-Rh(D) immunoglobulin

Is hydrops present?

No
• Management depends on gestational age, severity, fetal well-being, and likely etiology
• Consider MFM, NICU consultation
• Antenatal steroids, if indicated
• Serial ultrasound examinations biweekly to evaluate fetal well-being, follow fetal growth, and **MCA Doppler velocimetry[6]**

Normal MCA Dopplers
• Continue expectant management
• **Serial MCA Doppler velocimetry measurements**

Elevated MCA Dopplers
• **Consider delivery versus PUBS and IUT[8]**
• **Serial MCA Doppler velocimetry measurements**

Yes
• Management depends on gestational age, severity, and likely etiology
• **Review management options with the couple (including pregnancy termination if prior to viability)**
• Consider MFM, NICU consultation
• **Antenatal steroids, if indicated**

• For moderate and severe hydrops, **consider immediate delivery regardless of gestational age vs PUBS and IUT[8]**
• Serial ultrasound examinations with MCA Doppler velocimetry

1. Isoimmunization occurs when fetal erythrocytes express a protein(s) which is not present on maternal erythrocytes. Since there is constant trafficking of fetal cells across the placenta into the maternal circulation, the maternal immune system can become sensitized and produce antibodies against these "foreign" proteins. Maternal IgG antibodies can cross the placenta and destroy fetal erythrocytes, leading to fetal anemia and high-output cardiac failure, known as immune hydrops fetalis. Immune hydrops is associated with a fetal hematocrit <15% (normal 50%). The most antigenic protein on the surface of erythrocytes is D, also known as rhesus D or (Rh)D. Other antigens which can cause severe immune hydrops include Kell ("Kell kills"), Rh-E, Rh-c, and Duffy ("Duffy dies"). Antigens causing

Obstetric Clinical Algorithms: Management and Evidence. By © E.R. Norwitz, M. Belfort, G.R. Saade and H. Miller.
Published 2010 Blackwell Publishing.

less severe hydrops include ABO, Rh-e, Rh-C, Fya, Ce, k, and s. Lewis[a,b] incompatibility can cause mild anemia but not hydrops ("Lewis lives") because they are primarily IgM antibodies.

2. Since the introduction of anti-(Rh)D immunoglobulin, 60% of immune hydrops is due to ABO incompatibility which cannot be prevented.

3. Hydrops fetalis (Latin for "edema of the fetus") is a radiologic diagnosis requiring the presence of an abnormal accumulation of fluid in more than one fetal extravascular compartment, including ascites, pericardial effusion, pleural effusion, subcutaneous edema or placental edema. Polyhydramnios is seen in 50–75% of cases. It is a rare but very serious complication of pregnancy with a high perinatal mortality (>50%). Of all cases of fetal hydrops, 90% are due to a nonimmune cause and 10% have an immune etiology. Nonimmune hydrops may be due to fetal cardiac abnormalities (20–35%), chromosomal anomalies such as Turner syndrome (15%), hematologic aberrations such as α-thalassemia (10%), and other causes (infections such as CMV or parvovirus B19, twin-to-twin transfusion, vascular malformations, placental anomalies, congenital metabolic disorders); 50–60% have no clear explanation.

4. If the father of the baby is Rh(D) negative, then the fetus must be Rh(D) negative and Rh(D) sensitization will not occur. However, because of the well-documented 10% likelihood of nonpaternity in a clinic population, anti-(Rh)D immunoglobulin is often still recommended. Amniocentesis can be performed to confirm fetal Rh(D) status. A more recent development is the use of maternal blood to determine fetal Rh(D) status, but this test remains investigational.

5. Exposure of Rh(D)-negative women to as little as 0.25 mL of Rh(D)-positive blood may induce an antibody response. Since the initial immune response is IgM (which does not cross the placenta), the index pregnancy is rarely affected. However, immunization in subsequent pregnancies will trigger an IgG response which will cross the placenta and cause hemolysis. Risk factors for Rh(D) sensitization include mismatched blood transfusion (95% sensitization rate), pregnancy (16–18% sensitization rate following normal pregnancy without anti-Rh(D) IgG, 1.3% with anti-Rh(D) IgG at delivery, 0.13% with anti-Rh(D) IgG at delivery and empirically at 28 weeks), abortion (3–6%), CVS/amniocentesis (1–3%), and ectopic pregnancy (<1%). Passive immunization with anti-Rh(D) IgG can destroy fetal erythrocytes before they evoke a maternal immune response. Anti-Rh(D) IgG should be given within 72 hours of potential exposure. 300μg (US) or 500 IU (UK) given intramuscularly will cover up to 30 mL of fetal whole blood or 15 mL of fetal red blood cells.

6. Immune-mediated fetal hemolysis results in release of bile pigment into amniotic fluid that can be measured as the change in optical density at wavelength 450 nm (ΔOD_{450}). Traditionally, the degree of hemolysis was measured by serial amniocentesis every 1–2 weeks starting in the mid second trimester. Amniotic fluid ΔOD_{450} measurements were then plotted against gestational age (Liley curve) in an attempt to predict fetal outcome. If the ΔOD_{450} rose into the upper 80% of zone 2 or into zone 3 of the Liley curve, prompt intervention was indicated. However, this test has been replaced almost entirely with noninvasive measurements of peak velocity in the middle cerebral artery (MCA) of the fetus using Doppler velocimetry. An elevated MCA peak velocity for gestational age has been shown to accurately identify fetuses with severe anemia requiring intervention.

7. Unlike ABO, the (Rh)D antigen is expressed only on primate erythrocytes. It is evident by 38 days of intrauterine life. Mutation in the D gene on chromosome 1 results in lack of expression of D antigen on circulating erythrocytes. Such individuals are regarded as Rh(D) negative. This mutation arose first in the Basque region of Spain, and the difference in prevalence of Rh(D)-negative individuals between the races may reflect the amount of Spanish blood in their ancestry: Caucasians, 15%; African-Americans, 8%; African, 4%; Native American, 1%; and Asian, 1%.

8. Percutaneous umbilical blood sampling (PUBS) involves ultrasound-guided aspiration of fetal blood from the umbilical cord. Advantages include the ability to obtain a rapid fetal karyotype and to measure several hematologic, immunologic, and acid–base parameters in the fetus. Intrauterine fetal blood transfusions (IUT) can also be performed, but have a procedure-related fetal loss rate of 1–5% and are therefore rarely performed after 32–34 weeks.

42 Macrosomia

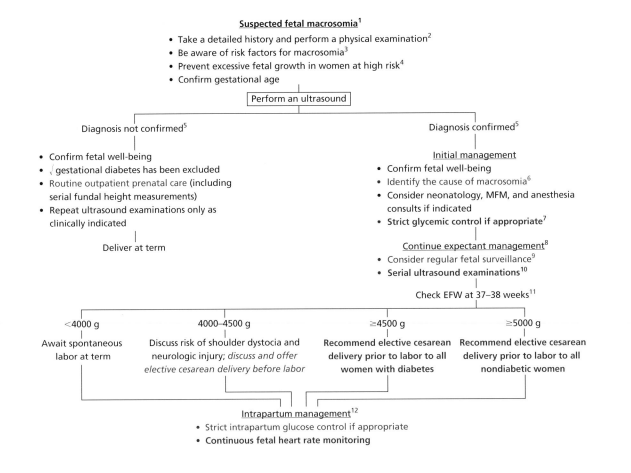

Suspected fetal macrosomia[1]
- Take a detailed history and perform a physical examination[2]
- Be aware of risk factors for macrosomia[3]
- Prevent excessive fetal growth in women at high risk[4]
- Confirm gestational age

Perform an ultrasound

Diagnosis not confirmed[5]
- Confirm fetal well-being
- √ gestational diabetes has been excluded
- Routine outpatient prenatal care (including serial fundal height measurements)
- Repeat ultrasound examinations only as clinically indicated

Deliver at term

Diagnosis confirmed[5]

Initial management
- Confirm fetal well-being
- Identify the cause of macrosomia[6]
- Consider neonatology, MFM, and anesthesia consults if indicated
- **Strict glycemic control if appropriate[7]**

Continue expectant management[8]
- Consider regular fetal surveillance[9]
- **Serial ultrasound examinations[10]**

Check EFW at 37–38 weeks[11]

<4000 g	4000–4500 g	≥4500 g	≥5000 g
Await spontaneous labor at term	Discuss risk of shoulder dystocia and neurologic injury; *discuss and offer elective cesarean delivery before labor*	Recommend elective cesarean delivery prior to labor to all women with diabetes	Recommend elective cesarean delivery prior to labor to all nondiabetic women

Intrapartum management[12]
- Strict intrapartum glucose control if appropriate
- **Continuous fetal heart rate monitoring**

1. Fetal macrosomia is defined most commonly as an estimated fetal weight (EFW) – not birthweight – of ≥4500 g (10 lb 8 oz). It is a single cut-off independent of gestational age or diabetic status. It should be distinguished from "large for gestational age" (LGA), which refers to a fetus with an EFW of >90th percentile for gestational age. Macrosomic fetuses have an increased risk of intrauterine and neonatal death as well as birth trauma, especially shoulder dystocia

and resultant neurologic (brachial plexus) injury. Other neonatal complications include hypoglycemia, polycythemia, hypocalcemia, and jaundice. In developing countries, 5% of infants weigh >4000 g at delivery and 0.5% weigh >4500 g.

2. The clinical diagnosis of fetal macrosomia is difficult, and physical examination alone will fail to identify over 50% of such fetuses. If the fundal height measurement is

Obstetric Clinical Algorithms: Management and Evidence. By © E.R. Norwitz, M. Belfort, G.R. Saade and H. Miller.
Published 2010 Blackwell Publishing.

significantly greater than expected ($>$3–4 cm for gestational age), an ultrasound examination should be performed.

3. Although a number of factors have been associated with fetal macrosomia, most women with risk factors have normal-weight babies. Risk factors include: (i) maternal diabetes (seen in 35–40% of macrosomic infants); (ii) post-term pregnancy (10–20%) – of all pregnancies continuing beyond 42 weeks' gestation, 2.5% are complicated by macrosomia; (iii) maternal obesity defined as a pre-pregnancy BMI $>$30 kg/m^2 (10–20%) – moreover, clinical and ultrasound estimation of fetal weight is far more difficult and less accurate in obese women; and (iv) other risk factors (such as multiparity, a prior macrosomic infant, a male infant, increased maternal height, advanced maternal age, and Beckwith–Wiedemann syndrome (pancreatic islet cell hyperplasia)).

4. Meticulous glycemic control throughout pregnancy in women with pregestational or gestational diabetes mellitus (GDM) can effectively reduce the incidence of fetal macrosomia.

5. Clinical estimation of fetal weight based on fundal height measurements and abdominal palpation (Leopold's maneuvers) is largely subjective, poorly reproducible, and depends on the experience of the obstetric care provider. It is especially unreliable in women with uterine fibroids and obesity, and in multiple pregnancies. For all these reasons, ultrasound is often used to estimate fetal weight. It should be noted, however, that ultrasound is accurate only to within 15–20% of actual fetal weight. Indeed, studies have shown that ultrasound is no more accurate in predicting actual fetal weight than a clinical examination by an experienced obstetrician or indeed than the estimate of the mother, providing she has had a previous child.

6. Most cases of macrosomia have no known cause. A detailed perinatal ultrasound should be performed to confirm gestational age, exclude other causes of a large fundal height (twins, fibroids, polyhydramnios), and to identify any fetal structural anomalies. In all cases, GDM should be excluded.

7. In women with GDM, the goal of antepartum management is to maintain strict glycemic control throughout gestation, defined as fasting blood glucose <95 mg/dL and 1 hour postprandial <140 mg/dL. This is typically achieved through a diabetic diet, moderate exercise, four times daily glucose monitoring, and additional treatment (insulin, oral hypoglycemic agents) as needed.

8. Because of the association between fetal macrosomia and birth trauma as well as peripartum maternal complications (including cesarean delivery, postpartum hemorrhage, severe perineal trauma, and puerperal infection), early induction of labor is often recommended with a view to maximizing the probability of a vaginal delivery. However, induction of labor for so-called "impending macrosomia" does not decrease the cesarean delivery rate. As such, this approach should not be encouraged.

9. Although the benefit is unclear in the absence of diabetes, most authorities recommend regular fetal surveillance, including daily kickcounts and weekly or twice-weekly nonstress testing and/or biophysical profile.

10. Serial growth scans should be performed every 2–3 weeks. More regular ultrasound examinations may be indicated to document amniotic fluid volume.

11. To prevent birth trauma, elective (prophylactic) cesarean delivery should be offered before the onset of labor at or after 39 weeks to diabetic women with an EFW $>$ 4500 g and nondiabetic women with an EFW $>$ 5000 g. An elective delivery prior to 39 weeks requires confirmation of fetal lung maturity.

12. Because of the risk of shoulder dystocia, attempted vaginal delivery of a macrosomic infant should take place in a controlled fashion, with immediate access to anesthesia staff and a neonatal resuscitation team. It is prudent to avoid assisted vaginal delivery in this setting.

43 Oligohydramnios[1]

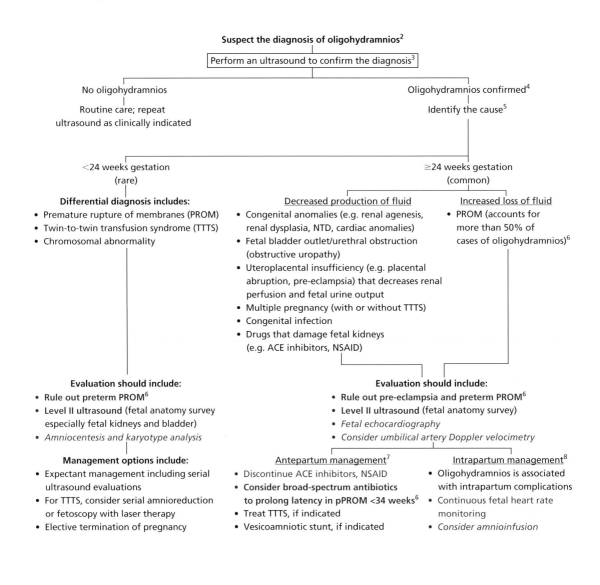

Suspect the diagnosis of oligohydramnios[2]

Perform an ultrasound to confirm the diagnosis[3]

No oligohydramnios

Routine care; repeat
ultrasound as clinically indicated

Oligohydramnios confirmed[4]

Identify the cause[5]

<24 weeks gestation
(rare)

≥24 weeks gestation
(common)

Differential diagnosis includes:
- Premature rupture of membranes (PROM)
- Twin-to-twin transfusion syndrome (TTTS)
- Chromosomal abnormality

Decreased production of fluid
- Congenital anomalies (e.g. renal agenesis,
  renal dysplasia, NTD, cardiac anomalies)
- Fetal bladder outlet/urethral obstruction
  (obstructive uropathy)
- Uteroplacental insufficiency (e.g. placental
  abruption, pre-eclampsia) that decreases renal
  perfusion and fetal urine output
- Multiple pregnancy (with or without TTTS)
- Congenital infection
- Drugs that damage fetal kidneys
  (e.g. ACE inhibitors, NSAID)

Increased loss of fluid
- PROM (accounts for
  more than 50% of
  cases of oligohydramnios)[6]

Evaluation should include:
- **Rule out preterm PROM[6]**
- **Level II ultrasound (fetal anatomy survey**
  especially fetal kidneys and bladder)
- *Amniocentesis and karyotype analysis*

Evaluation should include:
- **Rule out pre-eclampsia and preterm PROM[6]**
- **Level II ultrasound (fetal anatomy survey)**
- *Fetal echocardiography*
- *Consider umbilical artery Doppler velocimetry*

Management options include:
- Expectant management including serial
  ultrasound evaluations
- For TTTS, consider serial amnioreduction
  or fetoscopy with laser therapy
- Elective termination of pregnancy

Antepartum management[7]
- Discontinue ACE inhibitors, NSAID
- **Consider broad-spectrum antibiotics**
  to prolong latency in pPROM <34 weeks[6]
- Treat TTTS, if indicated
- Vesicoamniotic stunt, if indicated

Intrapartum management[8]
- Oligohydramnios is associated
  with intrapartum complications
- Continuous fetal heart rate
  monitoring
- *Consider amnioinfusion*

Obstetric Clinical Algorithms: Management and Evidence. By © E.R. Norwitz, M. Belfort, G.R. Saade and H. Miller.
Published 2010 Blackwell Publishing.

1. The amnion is a thin fetal membrane that begins to form on the eighth day postconception as a small sac covering the dorsal surface of the embryonic disk. The amnion gradually encircles the growing embryo. It is filled with amniotic fluid, which has a number of critical functions: (i) it cushions the fetus from external trauma; (ii) it protects the umbilical cord from excessive compression; (iii) it allows unrestricted fetal movement, thereby promoting the development of the fetal musculoskeletal system; (iv) it contributes to fetal pulmonary development; (v) it lubricates the fetal skin; (vi) it prevents maternal chorioamnionitis and fetal infection through its bacteriostatic properties; and (vii) it assists in fetal temperature control. Amniotic fluid volume is maximal at 34 weeks (750–800 mL) and decreases thereafter to 600 mL at 40 weeks. The amount of fluid continues to decrease beyond 40 weeks. Amniotic fluid volume is a marker of fetal well-being. Normal amniotic fluid volume suggests that uteroplacental perfusion is adequate. Oligohydramnios is associated with increased perinatal morbidity and mortality at any gestational age.

2. Oligohydramnios refers to an abnormally small amount of amniotic fluid surrounding the fetus. It is seen in 5–8% of all pregnancies. It should be suspected if the fundal height is significantly less than expected for gestational age.

3. Ultrasonography is a more accurate method of estimating amniotic fluid than measurement of fundal height. Several ultrasound techniques are described, including: (i) subjective assessment of amniotic fluid volume; (ii) measurement of the single deepest pocket (free of umbilical cord); (iii) Amniotic Fluid Index (AFI), which is a semi-quantitative method for estimating amniotic fluid volume which minimizes inter- and intraobserver error. AFI refers to the sum of the maximum vertical pocket of amniotic fluid (in cm) in each of the four quadrants of the uterus. Normal AFI beyond 20 weeks' gestation ranges from 5 to 20 cm.

4. Oligohydramnios is an ultrasound diagnosis. It is defined sonographically in a singleton pregnancy as a total amniotic fluid volume <300 mL, absence of a single vertical pocket ≥2 cm, or an AFI measurement <5th percentile for gestational age or <5 cm at term. In twins, absence of a single vertical pocket ≥2 cm is used to define oligohydramnios.

5. Maintenance of amniotic fluid volume is a dynamic process that reflects a balance between fluid production and absorption. Prior to 8 weeks' gestation, amniotic fluid is produced by passage of fluid across the amnion and fetal skin (transudation). At 8 weeks, the fetus begins to urinate into the amniotic cavity. Fetal urine quickly becomes the primary source of amniotic fluid production. Near term, 800–1000 mL of fetal urine is produced each day. The fetal lungs produce some fluid (300 mL per day at term), but much of it is swallowed before entering the amniotic space. Prior to 8 weeks' gestation, transudative amniotic fluid is passively reabsorbed. At 8 weeks' gestation, the fetus begins to swallow. Fetal swallowing quickly becomes the primary source of amniotic fluid absorption. Near term, 500–1000 mL of fluid is absorbed each day by fetal swallowing. A lesser amount of amniotic fluid is absorbed through the fetal membranes and enters the fetal bloodstream. Near term, 250 mL of amniotic fluid is absorbed by this route every day. Small quantities of amniotic fluid cross the amnion and enter the maternal bloodstream (10 mL per day near term). Every effort should be made to identify the cause of oligohydramnios. However, no cause will be found in approximately 30% of cases.

6. See Chapter 53.

7. The effect of oligohydramnios on the fetus depends on severity, gestational age, and underlying cause. Pulmonary hypoplasia, musculoskeletal deformities due to uterine compression (such as clubfoot), and/or amniotic band syndrome (adhesions between amnion and fetus causing serious deformities, including limb amputation) may develop in some cases. Antepartum treatment options are limited, unless a structural defect (such as an obstructive posterior urethral valve in a male infant) is identified and is amenable to *in utero* surgical repair or shunting.

8. The timing of delivery depends on gestational age, etiology, and fetal well-being. During labor, oligohydramnios is associated with an increased risk of nonreassuring fetal testing and cesarean delivery. Infusion of crystalloid solution into the amniotic cavity (amnioinfusion) may improve abnormal fetal heart rate patterns, decrease cesarean delivery rate, and (possibly) minimize the risk of neonatal meconium aspiration syndrome.

44 Recurrent Pregnancy Loss

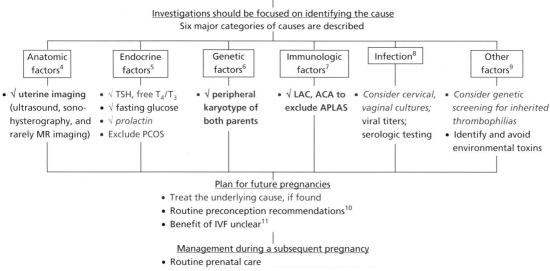

- Confirm the diagnosis[1]
- Take a detailed history and perform a physical examination[2]
- Consider differential diagnosis of recurrent pregnancy loss[3]

Investigations should be focused on identifying the cause
Six major categories of causes are described

Anatomic factors[4]	Endocrine factors[5]	Genetic factors[6]	Immunologic factors[7]	Infection[8]	Other factors[9]
• √ uterine imaging (ultrasound, sono-hysterography, and rarely MR imaging)	• √ TSH, free T$_4$/T$_3$ • √ fasting glucose • √ prolactin • Exclude PCOS	• √ peripheral karyotype of both parents	• √ LAC, ACA to exclude APLAS	• Consider cervical, vaginal cultures; viral titers; serologic testing	• Consider genetic screening for inherited thrombophilias • Identify and avoid environmental toxins

Plan for future pregnancies
- Treat the underlying cause, if found
- Routine preconception recommendations[10]
- Benefit of IVF unclear[11]

Management during a subsequent pregnancy
- Routine prenatal care
- Serial ultrasounds for fetal well-being and growth
- Consider delivery at 39–40 weeks

1. Recurrent pregnancy loss (RPL) is defined as the occurrence of three or more unexplained spontaneous early pregnancy losses before 20 weeks of gestation. These losses need not be consecutive. This condition occurs in approximately 1% of reproductive-age women.

2. Couples should ideally be seen prior to pregnancy. The pattern, trimester, and characteristics of the prior pregnancy losses should be reviewed. Exposure to environmental toxins/drugs, and prior gynecologic or obstetric infections should be specifically enquired about. A genetic pedigree should be developed and the possibility of consanguinity investigated. Physical examination may reveal evidence of maternal systemic disease or uterine

anomalies. Laboratory tests and imaging studies should be individualized.

3. The differential diagnosis of RPL can be divided into six categories (discussed below). Unfortunately, many couples (>50%) will have no identifiable cause even after extensive investigation. Informative and supportive counseling serves an important role. Couples are often anxious, frustrated, and on the verge of despair. This can lead to anxious patients and/or physicians exploring empiric or alternative treatments that have dubious benefit. Fortunately, the prognosis of unexplained RPL is good, and 60–70% of couples will have a subsequent healthy pregnancy even in the absence of any obstetric intervention.

Obstetric Clinical Algorithms: Management and Evidence. By © E.R. Norwitz, M. Belfort, G.R. Saade and H. Miller.
Published 2010 Blackwell Publishing.

4. <u>Anatomic factors</u> (account for 10–15% of cases of RPL). Congenital uterine anomalies resulting from Mullerian fusion abnormalities (such as didelphys or septate uterus) are most often associated with second-trimester losses. Surgical revision may be helpful in some cases. Cervical insufficiency also affects second-trimester losses, although this is regarded largely as a functional rather than a structural defect. Elective (prophylactic) cervical cerclage placement may be beneficial in selected patients.

5. <u>Endocrine factors</u> (10–15% of cases). Metabolic disorders (hypothyroidism, diabetes, polycyctic ovarian syndrome (PCOS)) require diagnosis and treatment of the underlying disease. Luteal phase deficiency is purported to result from insufficient progesterone secretion by the corpus luteum resulting in inadequate preparation of the endometrium for implantation and/or an inability to maintain early pregnancy, although the existence of such a diagnosis remains speculative. Two "out-of-phase" endometrial biopsies (in which histologic dating lags behind menstrual dating by ≥ 2 days) in consecutive cycles are required for the diagnosis. Progesterone supplementation is commonly prescribed, but without proven benefit.

6. <u>Genetic factors</u> (5–10% of cases). Abnormal parental chromosomal abnormalities are the only proven cause of RPL. The most frequent karyotypic abnormality is a balanced translocation and is found most often in the female partner: two-thirds are reciprocal (exchange of chromatin between any two nonhomologous chromosomes without loss of genetic material) and one-third are Robertsonian (fusion of chromosomes that have the centromere very near one end of a chromosome, typically 13, 14, 15, 21, or 22, with loss of one centromere and two short arms). The overall risk of spontaneous miscarriage in couples with a balanced translocation is >25%. Recurrent embryonic aneuploidy may represent nonrandom events in some predisposed couples. Most aneuploid losses are the result of advanced maternal age. Prenatal diagnosis via amniocentesis or chorionic villus sampling may be useful in some situations to facilitate diagnosis, but no treatment is available.

7. <u>Immunologic factors</u> (5–10% of cases). Antiphospholipid antibody syndrome (APLAS) is an autoimmune disorder characterized by circulating antibodies against membrane phospholipids and at least one specific clinical syndrome (RPL, unexplained thrombosis, autoimmune thrombocytopenia). The diagnosis requires at least one confirmatory serologic test (lupus anticoagulant (LAC) or anticardiolipin antibody (ACA)). The treatment is aspirin plus heparin. Alloimmunity (immunologic differences between individuals) has been proposed as a factor between reproductive partners that may cause RPL. During normal pregnancy, the mother's immune system is thought to recognize semi-allogeneic (50% "nonself") fetal antigens and to produce "blocking" factors to protect the fetus. Failure to produce these blocking factors may play a role, but there is no direct scientific evidence to support this theory and there is no specific diagnostic test. Immunotherapy has been used in an attempt to promote immune tolerance to paternal antigen, but has no proven benefit.

8. <u>Infection</u> (5% of cases). *Listeria monocytogenes, Mycoplasma hominis, Ureaplasma urealyticum, Toxoplasma gondii* and viruses (herpes simplex, cytomegalovirus, rubella) have been variously associated with spontaneous abortion, but none has been proven to cause RPL. Diagnosis can be made using cervical cultures, viral titers or serum antibodies. Directed antibiotic therapy may be useful if a causative agent is identified. Empiric treatment prior to pregnancy with doxycycline or erythromycin is more cost-effective, but is of unclear benefit.

9. <u>Other factors</u>. (i) Inherited thrombophilias may increase the risk of RPL, especially the factor V Leiden and prothrombin G2010A gene mutations. Anticoagulation may improve the chances of carrying a pregnancy to term. (ii) Environmental toxins such as smoking, alcohol, and heavy coffee consumption have been associated with spontaneous miscarriage, but not RPL. Regardless, use should be curtailed if possible. (iii) Drugs such as folic acid antagonists, valproic acid, warfarin, anesthetic gases, tetrachloroethylene, and isotretinoin (Accutane) are also speculative causes.

10. Routine preconception counseling includes avoidance of all alcohol consumption and prenatal vitamin supplementation including folic acid 1 mg daily.

11. *In vitro* fertilization (IVF) with or without preimplantation genetic diagnosis is often recommended for couples with RPL. With the possible exception of IVF with donor gametes in couples with documented genetic disorders (such as a parental balanced translocation), IVF is of unclear benefit in this setting.

45 Placenta Accreta

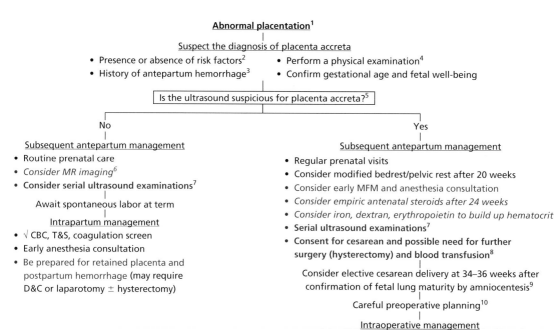

Abnormal placentation[1]

Suspect the diagnosis of placenta accreta

- Presence or absence of risk factors[2]
- History of antepartum hemorrhage[3]
- Perform a physical examination[4]
- Confirm gestational age and fetal well-being

Is the ultrasound suspicious for placenta accreta?[5]

No

Subsequent antepartum management
- Routine prenatal care
- *Consider MR imaging[6]*
- **Consider serial ultrasound examinations[7]**

Await spontaneous labor at term

Intrapartum management
- √ CBC, T&S, coagulation screen
- Early anesthesia consultation
- Be prepared for retained placenta and postpartum hemorrhage (may require D&C or laparotomy ± hysterectomy)

Yes

Subsequent antepartum management
- Regular prenatal visits
- Consider modified bedrest/pelvic rest after 20 weeks
- Consider early MFM and anesthesia consultation
- *Consider empiric antenatal steroids after 24 weeks*
- *Consider iron, dextran, erythropoietin to build up hematocrit*
- **Serial ultrasound examinations[7]**
- **Consent for cesarean and possible need for further surgery (hysterectomy) and blood transfusion[8]**

Consider elective cesarean delivery at 34–36 weeks after confirmation of fetal lung maturity by amniocentesis[9]

Careful preoperative planning[10]

Intraoperative management
- √ CBC, coagulation screen, T&S, large-bore iv access
- *Consider preoperative internal iliac artery balloon catheters*
- Early and aggressive fluid and blood product resuscitation
- Consider midline vertical skin incision, high vertical ("classic") hysterotomy, immediate closure of hysterotomy (do not remove placenta!) and puerperal hysterectomy

1. Abnormal placentation refers to an abnormal attachment of the placental villi to the underlying maternal tissues of the uterus. These conditions can be divided into: (i) placenta accreta (80%) in which the placental villi invade abnormally into the myometrium, (ii) placenta increta (15%) in which the placental villi invade abnormally through the myometrium but not through the serosa, and (iii) placenta percreta (5%) in which the placental villi invade through the myometrium, through the serosa, and into the surrounding tissues including the bladder, bowel or broad ligament. Of these, placenta accreta is the most common type and complicates 1 in 2500 deliveries.

2. Risk factors for placenta accreta include prior uterine surgery (such as cesarean delivery, myomectomy, D&C, hysteroscopic resection), placenta previa, advanced maternal age, smoking, and grand multiparity (defined as >5

Obstetric Clinical Algorithms: Management and Evidence. By © E.R. Norwitz, M. Belfort, G.R. Saade and H. Miller.
Published 2010 Blackwell Publishing.

prior deliveries). Placenta previa alone is associated with a 5% incidence of accreta, which increases to 15–20% with placenta previa and one prior cesarean and >50% with placenta previa and two or more prior cesareans. An unexplained elevation in maternal serum α-fetoprotein (MS-AFP) at 15–20 weeks' gestation is also associated with abnormal placentation.

3. Most women with placenta accreta do not develop symptoms during pregnancy. However, some women may present with acute onset of bright-red vaginal bleeding, which is usually painless. This is most common if there is an accompanying placenta previa. Abdominal pain is rare. Other causes of antepartum hemorrhage include placenta previa alone (see Chapter 46), placental abruption (Chapter 47), vasa previa (Chapter 67), early labor, and genital tract lesions (cervical polyps or erosions). Bleeding is of maternal origin. If excessive, it can lead to hemodynamic instability and shock.

4. Physical examination is usually unhelpful. When a woman presents with antepartum hemorrhage, pelvic examination should be avoided until placenta previa is excluded on ultrasound. In the setting of placenta previa, fetal malpresentation is common.

5. There are four major sonographic features of placenta accreta: (i) loss of the hypoechoic zone between the uterus and the bladder, (ii) loss of the smooth interface with the bladder, (iii) "Swiss cheese" appearance (vascular lacunae) within the placenta, and (iv) focal nodular projections beyond the uterus and typically into the bladder. Color flow imaging may show chaotic blood flow between the placenta and bladder or pulsatile flow within the bladder wall. Placenta accreta may be an incidental finding on routine ultrasound.

6. If the ultrasound examination is equivocal, consider magnetic resonance (MR) imaging. Initial studies suggested that MR imaging was more sensitive than ultrasound in diagnosing placenta accreta, but recent studies have found no difference between the two modalities (with a sensitivity of approximately 50%). MR imaging may be particularly useful for posterior previa, a situation in which ultrasound is more limited.

7. Serial ultrasound examinations may be useful to follow placental location, fetal presentation, fetal growth, and sonographic markers of placenta accreta.

8. The goal of antepartum management in the setting of placenta accreta is to maximize fetal maturation while minimizing risk to mother and fetus. Nonreassuring fetal testing ("fetal distress") and excessive maternal hemorrhage are contraindications to expectant management, and may necessitate immediate cesarean irrespective of gestational age. Contraindications to emergency cesarean include a previable fetus (<23–24 weeks), intrauterine fetal demise, maternal hemodynamic instability or uncontrolled coagulopathy, or failure to obtain maternal consent for surgery.

9. In the setting of suspected placenta accreta, vaginal delivery is rarely appropriate. Elective cesarean under controlled conditions prior to the onset of labor is optimal. However, vaginal delivery may be considered in the setting of intrauterine fetal demise, fetal malformations incompatible with life, advanced labor with engagement of the fetal head and minimal vaginal bleeding, or an indicated delivery with a previable fetus.

10. Careful preoperative planning is essential, and should include discussions with staff from anesthesia, OR, blood bank, urology, MFM, NICU, and possibly gynecologic oncology, vascular surgery, and interventional radiology. Consider mode of anesthesia (usually general endotracheal anesthesia and possible epidural for postoperative pain control), utility of central monitoring (arterial line, central venous line and/or Swan–Ganz catheter), preoperative cystoscopy and stenting of ureters, use of cell saver equipment and/or normovolemic hemodilution to minimize need for blood transfusion, adequate suction capacity, blood warmers, body warmers, and pneumatic compression stockings (for DVT prophylaxis).

46 Placenta Previa

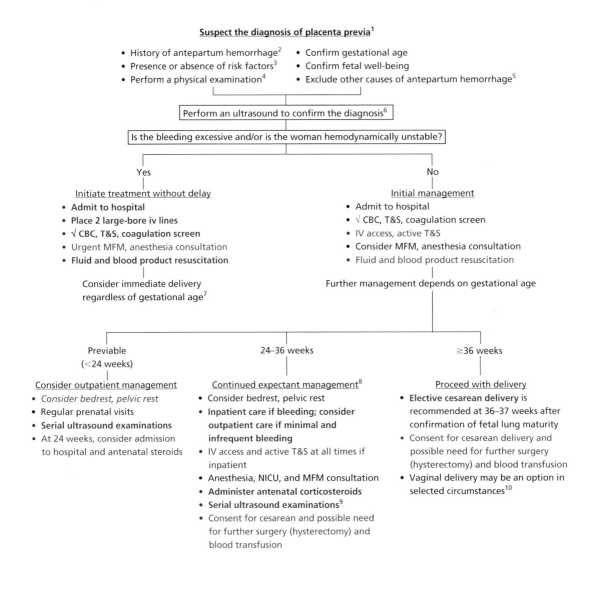

Suspect the diagnosis of placenta previa[1]

- History of antepartum hemorrhage[2]
- Presence or absence of risk factors[3]
- Perform a physical examination[4]

- Confirm gestational age
- Confirm fetal well-being
- Exclude other causes of antepartum hemorrhage[5]

Perform an ultrasound to confirm the diagnosis[6]

Is the bleeding excessive and/or is the woman hemodynamically unstable?

Yes

Initiate treatment without delay
- **Admit to hospital**
- **Place 2 large-bore iv lines**
- **√ CBC, T&S, coagulation screen**
- Urgent MFM, anesthesia consultation
- **Fluid and blood product resuscitation**

Consider immediate delivery regardless of gestational age[7]

No

Initial management
- **Admit to hospital**
- **√ CBC, T&S, coagulation screen**
- IV access, active T&S
- Consider MFM, anesthesia consultation
- Fluid and blood product resuscitation

Further management depends on gestational age

Previable
(<24 weeks)

Consider outpatient management
- *Consider bedrest, pelvic rest*
- Regular prenatal visits
- **Serial ultrasound examinations**
- At 24 weeks, consider admission to hospital and antenatal steroids

24–36 weeks

Continued expectant management[8]
- Consider bedrest, pelvic rest
- **Inpatient care if bleeding; consider outpatient care if minimal and infrequent bleeding**
- IV access and active T&S at all times if inpatient
- Anesthesia, NICU, and MFM consultation
- **Administer antenatal corticosteroids**
- **Serial ultrasound examinations[9]**
- Consent for cesarean and possible need for further surgery (hysterectomy) and blood transfusion

≥36 weeks

Proceed with delivery
- **Elective cesarean delivery** is recommended at 36–37 weeks after confirmation of fetal lung maturity
- Consent for cesarean delivery and possible need for further surgery (hysterectomy) and blood transfusion
- Vaginal delivery may be an option in selected circumstances[10]

Obstetric Clinical Algorithms: Management and Evidence. By © E.R. Norwitz, M. Belfort, G.R. Saade and H. Miller.
Published 2010 Blackwell Publishing.

1. Placenta previa refers to implantation of the placenta over the cervical os in advance of the fetal presenting part. It complicates 1 in 200 pregnancies, and accounts for 20% of all cases of antepartum hemorrhage.

2. Symptoms may include the acute onset of bright-red vaginal bleeding, which is usually painless. It is often accompanied by decreased fetal movement. Bleeding is of maternal origin. Fetal malpresentation is common, because the placenta prevents engagement of the presenting part. It may be an incidental finding on routine ultrasound.

3. Risk factors for placenta previa include multiparity, advanced maternal age, prior placenta previa, prior cesarean delivery, and smoking.

4. When a woman presents with antepartum hemorrhage, pelvic examination should be avoided until placenta previa is excluded on ultrasound.

5. Other causes of antepartum hemorrhage include placental abruption (see Chapter 47), vasa previa (see Chapter 67), early labor, and genital tract lesions (cervical polyps or erosions).

6. Placenta previa is an ultrasound diagnosis. Transperineal and/or transvaginal ultrasound may be necessary to confirm the diagnosis, and is regarded as safe in this setting. Of note, only 5% of placenta previa identified by ultrasound at routine second-trimester fetal anatomy survey will persist to term. Placenta accreta (abnormal attachment of placental villi to the uterine wall) is rare (1 in 2500 pregnancies), but complicates 5% of pregnancies with placenta previa, 10–25% with placenta previa and one prior cesarean, and >50% with placenta previa and two or more prior cesareans (see Chapter 45).

7. Emergency cesarean delivery may be needed. Contraindications to emergency cesarean include a previable fetus (<23–24 weeks), intrauterine fetal demise, maternal hemodynamic instability or uncontrolled coagulopathy, or failure to obtain maternal consent for surgery.

8. The goal of antepartum management in the setting of placenta previa is to maximize fetal maturation while minimizing risk to mother and fetus. Nonreassuring fetal testing ("fetal distress") and excessive maternal hemorrhage are contraindications to expectant management, and may necessitate immediate cesarean irrespective of gestational age. However, most episodes of bleeding are not life-threatening. With careful monitoring, delivery can be safely delayed in most cases. Outpatient management may be an option for women with a single small bleed if they can comply with restrictions on activity and maintain proximity to a hospital. Placenta previa may resolve with time, thereby permitting vaginal delivery.

9. Serial ultrasound examinations are useful to follow placental location, fetal presentation (malpresentation is common), and possibly fetal growth (although placenta previa is not associated with intrauterine growth restriction).

10. Vaginal delivery is rarely appropriate in the setting of placenta previa, but may be indicated in the setting of intrauterine fetal demise, fetal malformation(s) incompatible with life, advanced labor with engagement of the fetal head and minimal vaginal bleeding, or an indicated delivery with a previable fetus. A double set-up examination in labor may be appropriate when ultrasound cannot exclude placenta previa and the patient is strongly motivated for vaginal delivery. This procedure is performed in the operating room with surgical anesthesia and two surgical teams. One team is scrubbed and ready for immediate cesarean in the event of hemorrhage or nonreassuring fetal testing ("fetal distress"). The other team then performs a gentle bimanual examination initially of the vaginal fornices and then the cervical os. If a previa is present, immediate cesarean is indicated. If no placenta is palpated, amniotomy can be performed and labor induced.

47 Placental Abruption

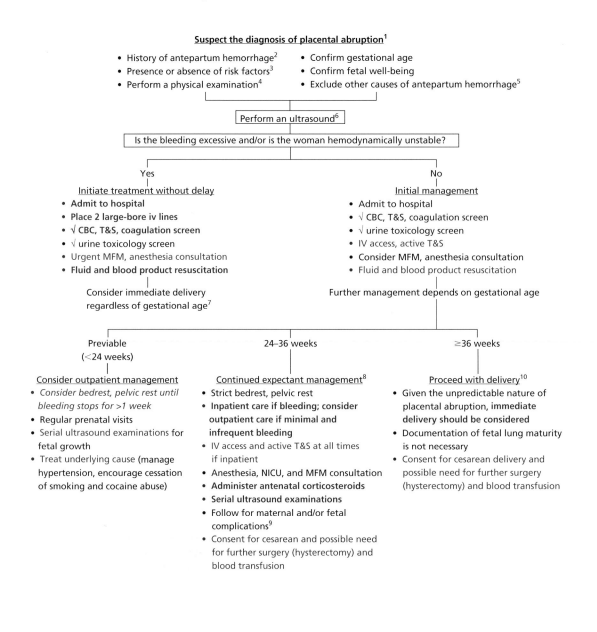

Suspect the diagnosis of placental abruption[1]

- History of antepartum hemorrhage[2]
- Presence or absence of risk factors[3]
- Perform a physical examination[4]
- Confirm gestational age
- Confirm fetal well-being
- Exclude other causes of antepartum hemorrhage[5]

Perform an ultrasound[6]

Is the bleeding excessive and/or is the woman hemodynamically unstable?

Yes

Initiate treatment without delay
- **Admit to hospital**
- **Place 2 large-bore iv lines**
- **√ CBC, T&S, coagulation screen**
- **√ urine toxicology screen**
- Urgent MFM, anesthesia consultation
- **Fluid and blood product resuscitation**

Consider immediate delivery
regardless of gestational age[7]

No

Initial management
- Admit to hospital
- √ CBC, T&S, coagulation screen
- √ urine toxicology screen
- IV access, active T&S
- Consider MFM, anesthesia consultation
- Fluid and blood product resuscitation

Further management depends on gestational age

Previable
(<24 weeks)

Consider outpatient management
- *Consider bedrest, pelvic rest until bleeding stops for >1 week*
- Regular prenatal visits
- Serial ultrasound examinations for fetal growth
- Treat underlying cause (manage hypertension, encourage cessation of smoking and cocaine abuse)

24–36 weeks

Continued expectant management[8]
- Strict bedrest, pelvic rest
- **Inpatient care if bleeding; consider outpatient care if minimal and infrequent bleeding**
- IV access and active T&S at all times if inpatient
- Anesthesia, NICU, and MFM consultation
- **Administer antenatal corticosteroids**
- **Serial ultrasound examinations**
- Follow for maternal and/or fetal complications[9]
- Consent for cesarean and possible need for further surgery (hysterectomy) and blood transfusion

≥36 weeks

Proceed with delivery[10]
- Given the unpredictable nature of placental abruption, **immediate delivery should be considered**
- Documentation of fetal lung maturity is not necessary
- Consent for cesarean delivery and possible need for further surgery (hysterectomy) and blood transfusion

Obstetric Clinical Algorithms: Management and Evidence. By © E.R. Norwitz, M. Belfort, G.R. Saade and H. Miller.
Published 2010 Blackwell Publishing.

1. Placental abruption refers to premature separation of the placenta from the uterine wall. The bleeding that results may be revealed vaginally (80%) or concealed within the uterus (20%). Abruption complicates 1 in 120 pregnancies, and accounts for 30% of all cases of antepartum hemorrhage.

2. Symptoms may include vaginal bleeding (80%), uterine contractions (35%), and abdominal tenderness (70%) with or without nonreassuring fetal testing (50%). Bleeding is of maternal origin. Uterine tenderness suggests extravasation of blood into the myometrium (Couvelaire uterus). The amount of vaginal bleeding may not be a reliable indicator of the severity of the hemorrhage since bleeding may be concealed. Serial measurements of fundal height and abdominal girth are useful to monitor large retroplacental blood collections. Rarely, placental abruption may be an incidental finding on routine ultrasound.

3. Risk factors for placental abruption include hypertension, prior placental abruption (recurrence rate is 10% after one abruption, 25% after two abruptions), trauma, smoking, cocaine, uterine anomaly or fibroids, multiparity, advanced maternal age, preterm premature rupture of the membranes, an inherited or acquired bleeding diathesis, and rapid decompression of an overdistended uterus (such as multiple pregnancy or polyhydramnios).

4. When a woman presents with antepartum hemorrhage, pelvic examination should be avoided until placenta previa is excluded on ultrasound.

5. Other causes of antepartum hemorrhage include placenta previa (see Chapter 46), vasa previa (see Chapter 67), early labor, and genital tract lesions (cervical polyps or erosions).

6. Placental abruption is a clinical diagnosis. An ultrasound should be performed to exclude placenta previa, confirm gestational age, document estimated fetal weight, and confirm fetal well-being. Since a retroplacental collection of ≥300 mL is necessary for sonographic visualization, only 2% of abruptions can be visualized on ultrasound. Port-wine discoloration of the amniotic fluid at the time of amniocentesis or cesarean delivery is highly suggestive of placental abruption.

7. Emergency cesarean delivery may be needed. Contraindications to emergency cesarean include a previable fetus (< 23–24 weeks), intrauterine fetal demise, maternal hemodynamic instability or uncontrolled coagulopathy, or failure to obtain maternal consent for surgery.

8. The goal of antepartum management is to maximize fetal maturation while minimizing risk to mother and fetus. Hospitalization is indicated to evaluate the maternal and fetal conditions. Nonreassuring fetal testing ("fetal distress") and excessive maternal hemorrhage are contraindications to expectant management, and may necessitate immediate cesarean irrespective of gestational age. However, most episodes of bleeding are not life-threatening. With careful monitoring, delivery can be safely delayed in most cases. Outpatient management may be an option if the bleeding is small and infrequent and if the woman can comply with restrictions on activity and maintain proximity to a hospital. Placental abruption is a relative contraindication to tocolysis. Serial ultrasound examinations are useful to follow the appearance of the placenta, fetal presentation, and fetal growth, and possibly umbilical artery Doppler velocimetry.

9. Maternal mortality ranges from 0.5% to 5% due to excessive hemorrhage, cardiac failure or renal failure. Clinically significant coagulopathy occurs in 10% of cases. Perinatal complications include intrauterine fetal demise in 10–35% of cases due to fetal hypoxia or exsanguination, and neonatal death due to complications of prematurity. Abruption is also associated with an increased rate of congenital anomalies and IUGR.

10. Mode and timing of delivery depend on the condition and gestational age of the fetus, condition of the mother and state of the cervix.

48 Polyhydramnios[1]

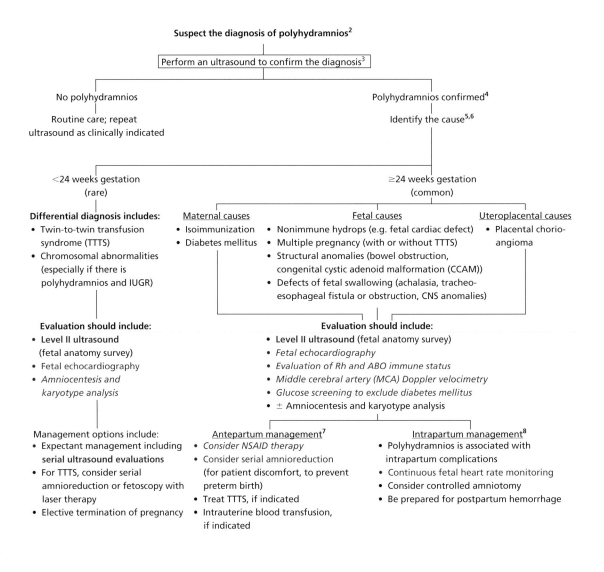

Suspect the diagnosis of polyhydramnios[2]

Perform an ultrasound to confirm the diagnosis[3]

No polyhydramnios

Routine care; repeat ultrasound as clinically indicated

Polyhydramnios confirmed[4]

Identify the cause[5,6]

<24 weeks gestation (rare)

≥24 weeks gestation (common)

Differential diagnosis includes:
- Twin-to-twin transfusion syndrome (TTTS)
- Chromosomal abnormalities (especially if there is polyhydramnios and IUGR)

Maternal causes
- Isoimmunization
- Diabetes mellitus

Fetal causes
- Nonimmune hydrops (e.g. fetal cardiac defect)
- Multiple pregnancy (with or without TTTS)
- Structural anomalies (bowel obstruction, congenital cystic adenoid malformation (CCAM))
- Defects of fetal swallowing (achalasia, tracheo-esophageal fistula or obstruction, CNS anomalies)

Uteroplacental causes
- Placental chorio-angioma

Evaluation should include:
- **Level II ultrasound** (fetal anatomy survey)
- Fetal echocardiography
- *Amniocentesis and karyotype analysis*

Evaluation should include:
- **Level II ultrasound** (fetal anatomy survey)
- *Fetal echocardiography*
- *Evaluation of Rh and ABO immune status*
- *Middle cerebral artery (MCA) Doppler velocimetry*
- *Glucose screening to exclude diabetes mellitus*
- ± Amniocentesis and karyotype analysis

Management options include:
- Expectant management including **serial ultrasound evaluations**
- For TTTS, consider serial amnioreduction or fetoscopy with laser therapy
- Elective termination of pregnancy

Antepartum management[7]
- *Consider NSAID therapy*
- Consider serial amnioreduction (for patient discomfort, to prevent preterm birth)
- Treat TTTS, if indicated
- Intrauterine blood transfusion, if indicated

Intrapartum management[8]
- Polyhydramnios is associated with intrapartum complications
- Continuous fetal heart rate monitoring
- Consider controlled amniotomy
- Be prepared for postpartum hemorrhage

Obstetric Clinical Algorithms: Management and Evidence. By © E.R. Norwitz, M. Belfort, G.R. Saade and H. Miller.
Published 2010 Blackwell Publishing.

1. The amnion is a thin fetal membrane that begins to form on the eighth day postconception as a small sac covering the dorsal surface of the embryonic disc. The amnion gradually encircles the growing embryo. It is filled with amniotic fluid which has a number of critical functions: (i) it cushions the fetus from external trauma; (ii) it protects the umbilical cord from excessive compression; (iii) it allows unrestricted fetal movement, thereby promoting the development of the fetal musculoskeletal system; (iv) it contributes to fetal pulmonary development; (v) it lubricates the fetal skin; (vi) it prevents maternal chorioamnionitis and fetal infection through its bacteriostatic properties; and (vii) it assists in fetal temperature control. Amniotic fluid volume is maximal at 34 weeks (750–800 mL) and decreases thereafter to 600 mL at 40 weeks. The amount of fluid continues to decrease beyond 40 weeks. Amniotic fluid volume is a marker of fetal well-being. Normal amniotic fluid volume suggests that utero-placental perfusion is adequate. Abnormal amount of amniotic fluid volume is associated with an unfavorable perinatal outcome.

2. Polyhydramnios refers to an abnormally large amount of amniotic fluid surrounding the fetus. It is seen in 0.5–1.5% of all pregnancies. It should be suspected if the fundal height is significantly more than expected for gestational age.

3. Ultrasonography is a more accurate method of estimating amniotic fluid than measurement of fundal height. Several ultrasound techniques are described, including: (i) subjective assessment of amniotic fluid volume; (ii) measurement of the single deepest pocket (free of umbilical cord); (iii) Amniotic Fluid Index (AFI), which is a semi-quantitative method for estimating amniotic fluid volume which minimizes inter- and intraobserver error. AFI refers to the sum of the maximum vertical pocket of amniotic fluid (in cm) in each of the four quadrants of the uterus. Normal AFI beyond 20 weeks' gestation ranges from 5 to 20 cm.

4. Polyhydramnios is an ultrasound diagnosis. It is defined sonographically in a singleton pregnancy as a total amniotic fluid volume >2 L, a single vertical pocket ≥10 cm or an AFI measurement >95th percentile for gestational age or >20 cm at term. In twins, a single vertical pocket ≥10 cm is used to defined polyhydramnios.

5. Maintenance of amniotic fluid volume is a dynamic process that reflects a balance between fluid production and absorption. Prior to 8 weeks' gestation, amniotic fluid is produced by passage of fluid across the amnion and fetal skin (transudation). At 8 weeks, the fetus begins to urinate into the amniotic cavity. Fetal urine quickly becomes the primary source of amniotic fluid production. Near term, 800–1000 mL of fetal urine is produced each day. The fetal lungs produce some fluid (300 mL per day at term), but much of it is swallowed before entering the amniotic space. Prior to 8 weeks' gestation, transudative amniotic fluid is passively reabsorbed. At 8 weeks' gestation, the fetus begins to swallow. Fetal swallowing quickly becomes the primary source of amniotic fluid absorption. Near term, 500–1000 mL of fluid is absorbed each day by fetal swallowing. A lesser amount of amniotic fluid is absorbed through the fetal membranes and enters the fetal bloodstream. Near term, 250 mL of amniotic fluid is absorbed by this route every day. Small quantities of amniotic fluid cross the amnion and enter the maternal bloodstream (10 mL per day near term).

6. Every effort should be made to identify the cause. However, no cause will be found in 50–60% of cases of polyhydramnios.

7. Uterine overdistension may result in maternal dyspnea or refractory edema of the lower extremities and vulva. It can also lead to preterm PROM as well as premature labor and delivery. Antepartum treatment options are limited. Nonsteroidal anti-inflammatory drugs (NSAID) (such as indomethacin) can decrease fetal urine production, but may cause premature closure of the ductus arteriosus *in utero*, leading to pulmonary hypertension. Removal of fluid by amniocentesis is only transiently effective as fluid will typically reaccumulate within 24–72 hours. Treatment of the underlying disorder (such as laser therapy for TTTS or intrauterine transfusion for pregnancies complicated by isoimmunization and severe fetal anemia) may reverse the polyhydramnios.

8. During labor, polyhydramnios can result in fetal malpresentation, dysfunctional labor, and/or postpartum hemorrhage. Controlled amniotomy may reduce the incidence of complications resulting from rapid decompression of the uterus (such as placental abruption and cord prolapse).

49 Post-term Pregnancy[1]

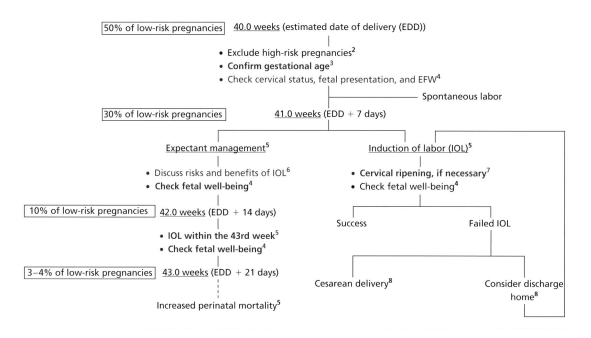

| 50% of low-risk pregnancies | 40.0 weeks (estimated date of delivery (EDD)) |

- Exclude high-risk pregnancies[2]
- **Confirm gestational age[3]**
- Check cervical status, fetal presentation, and EFW[4]

———————————————— Spontaneous labor

| 30% of low-risk pregnancies | 41.0 weeks (EDD + 7 days) |

Expectant management[5]

- Discuss risks and benefits of IOL[6]
- **Check fetal well-being[4]**

Induction of labor (IOL)[5]

- **Cervical ripening, if necessary[7]**
- Check fetal well-being[4]

Success   Failed IOL

| 10% of low-risk pregnancies | 42.0 weeks (EDD + 14 days) |

- IOL within the 43rd week[5]
- **Check fetal well-being[4]**

| 3–4% of low-risk pregnancies | 43.0 weeks (EDD + 21 days) |

Increased perinatal mortality[5]

Cesarean delivery[8]   Consider discharge home[8]

---

1. Post-term (prolonged) pregnancy refers to a pregnancy that has extended to or beyond a gestational age of 42.0 weeks (294 days) from the first day of the last menstrual period. The term "post dates" is poorly defined and should be avoided. An alternative and simpler approach is to date the pregnancy relative to the estimated date of delivery (EDD); 42.0 weeks would therefore be EDD + 14 days.

2. Delivery is typically recommended when the risks to the fetus of continuing the pregnancy are greater than those faced by the neonate after birth. High-risk pregnancies should not be allowed to go post-term because, in these pregnancies, the balance appears to shift in favor of delivery at around 38–39 weeks of gestation. This is true also of twin pregnancies. These guidelines therefore apply only to uncomplicated <u>low-risk</u> post-term pregnancies.

3. Accurate pregnancy dating is important in minimizing the false diagnosis of post-term pregnancy. The EDD is most reliably and accurately determined early in pregnancy. This may be based upon a known LMP in women with regular, normal menstrual cycles. Consistency between historical and physical data is important in establishing the reliability of dating. Other clinical data should be consistent with the EDD, as follows.

- The size of the uterus at early examination (in the first trimester) should be consistent with dates.
- The perception of fetal movement (quickening) usually occurs at 18–20 weeks in nulliparous women and 16–18 weeks in multiparous women.
- The fetal heart can be heard with a nonelectronic fetal stethoscope by 18–20 weeks in most patients.
- At 20 weeks, the fundal height should be approximately 20 cm above the symphysis pubis, which usually corresponds with the umbilicus.

Inconsistencies or concern about the accuracy of the dating require further assessment with ultrasonography. Useful measurements include the crown–rump length

---

Obstetric Clinical Algorithms: Management and Evidence. By © E.R. Norwitz, M. Belfort, G.R. Saade and H. Miller.
Published 2010 Blackwell Publishing.

of the fetus during the first trimester and the biparietal diameter or head circumference and femur length during the second trimester. Because of the normal variations in size of infants in the third trimester, dating the pregnancy at that time is less reliable (± 3 weeks).

4. Even though evidence of either a positive or negative effect is lacking, antenatal fetal surveillance for post-term pregnancies has become standard practice. Options for fetal surveillance include nonstress testing, biophysical profile (BPP) or modified BPP (amniotic fluid volume estimation), the oxytocin challenge test or a combination of these modalities. No single method has been shown to be superior. Of note, Doppler velocimetry has no proven benefit in monitoring the post-term fetus and is not recommended for this indication. Although no firm recommendation can be made regarding the frequency of antenatal surveillance among post-term patients, many experts would advise twice-weekly testing with some evaluation of amniotic fluid volume performed at least weekly. Delivery should be effected immediately if there is evidence of fetal compromise or oligohydramnios. There is insufficient evidence to show that initiating antenatal surveillance at 40–42 weeks improves pregnancy outcome or confers any benefit to the fetus.

5. At 41 weeks (EDD + 7 days), both expectant management and induction of labor are associated with low complication rates and good perinatal outcomes in low-risk post-term gravida. Since delivery cannot always be brought about readily, maternal risks and considerations are apt to confound this decision. Factors that need to be considered include gestational age, results of antepartum fetal testing, favorability of the cervix, and maternal preference after discussion of the risks and benefits of the management options. According to current obstetric practice, labor is generally induced when the cervix is favorable, as the risk of failed induction and subsequent cesarean delivery is low. If the cervix is unfavorable, the optimal approach is less clear. Even if the cervix is unfavorable, there appears to be a small advantage to induction of labor, regardless of parity or method of induction.

However, expectant management is a reasonable alternative in this setting.

6. ACOG has no specific recommendations about the timing of delivery. However, most authorities would recommend IOL for all low-risk pregnancies sometime during the 43rd week of gestation, because of the increased risk to the fetus of continuing the pregnancy. These include an increase in perinatal mortality, uteroplacental insufficiency (chronic IUGR leading to "fetal dysmaturity syndrome"), fetal macrosomia (which is associated with prolonged labor, cephalopelvic disproportion, and shoulder dystocia with resultant risks of orthopedic or neurologic injury), and asphyxia (with and without meconium). In addition to the risks to the fetus, post-term pregnancy is also associated with risks to the mother including an increase in labor dystocia, severe perineal injury, and a doubling in the rate of cesarean delivery.

7. The introduction of preinduction cervical maturation has resulted in fewer failed and serial inductions, lower fetal and maternal morbidity, a shorter hospital stay, and possibly a lower rate of cesarean delivery in the general obstetric population. Both PGE2 (dinoprostone) and PGE1 (misoprostol) have been used for IOL in post-term pregnancies. Although the dose, dosage interval, route of administration, and side-effect profile vary slightly between the different preparations, these agents appear to be equally effective. Overall, these medications are well tolerated with few reported side-effects. Higher doses of prostaglandins have been associated with an increased risk of uterine tachysystole and hyperstimulation leading to non-reassuring fetal testing. As such, lower doses are preferable. Given the risk of uterine hyperstimulation, postapplication fetal heart rate monitoring should be carried out routinely to ensure fetal well-being.

8. The decision of whether to proceed with cesarean delivery or discharge the patient home in the setting of failed IOL should be individualized. Factors that need to be considered include the precise gestational age, results of antepartum fetal testing, and maternal preference.

50 Prenatal Diagnosis

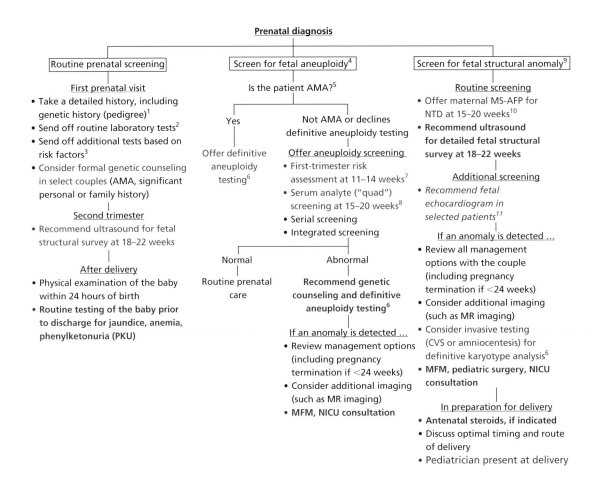

Prenatal diagnosis

Routine prenatal screening

First prenatal visit
- Take a detailed history, including genetic history (pedigree)[1]
- Send off routine laboratory tests[2]
- Send off additional tests based on risk factors[3]
- Consider formal genetic counseling in select couples (AMA, significant personal or family history)

Second trimester
- Recommend ultrasound for fetal structural survey at 18–22 weeks

After delivery
- Physical examination of the baby within 24 hours of birth
- **Routine testing of the baby prior to discharge for jaundice, anemia, phenylketonuria (PKU)**

Screen for fetal aneuploidy[4]

Is the patient AMA?[5]

Yes

Offer definitive aneuploidy testing[6]

Not AMA or declines definitive aneuploidy testing

Offer aneuploidy screening
- First-trimester risk assessment at 11–14 weeks[7]
- Serum analyte ("quad") screening at 15–20 weeks[8]
- Serial screening
- Integrated screening

Normal

Routine prenatal care

Abnormal

Recommend genetic counseling and definitive aneuploidy testing[6]

If an anomaly is detected …
- Review management options (including pregnancy termination if <24 weeks)
- Consider additional imaging (such as MR imaging)
- **MFM, NICU consultation**

Screen for fetal structural anomaly[9]

Routine screening
- Offer maternal MS-AFP for NTD at 15–20 weeks[10]
- **Recommend ultrasound for detailed fetal structural survey at 18–22 weeks**

Additional screening
- *Recommend fetal echocardiogram in selected patients[11]*

If an anomaly is detected …
- Review all management options with the couple (including pregnancy termination if <24 weeks)
- Consider additional imaging (such as MR imaging)
- Consider invasive testing (CVS or amniocentesis) for definitive karyotype analysis[6]
- **MFM, pediatric surgery, NICU consultation**

In preparation for delivery
- **Antenatal steroids, if indicated**
- Discuss optimal timing and route of delivery
- Pediatrician present at delivery

1. Ask about prior pregnancies, underlying medical conditions, personal and family history, and medication/drug exposure. Patient history may identify a fetus at risk for aneuploidy (genetic anomalies) or structural anomalies.

2. Routine testing at first prenatal visit includes: CBC, T&S, RPR, rubella serology, hepatitis B serology, HIV, PAP smear, PPD, cervical cultures (gonorrhea, chlamydia), and urinalysis. Toxoplasmosis, varicella, CMV, urine toxicology,

and TSH screening are not routinely recommended. All pregnant women should be offered genetic screening for cystic fibrosis carrier status (although the test is most reliable in Caucasian couples with a risk of 1/25). In the late second trimester, additional screening tests are recommended: repeat CBC, T&S, RPR, and urinalysis. Consider repeat HIV in high-risk couples (Chapter 27). Screening for gestational diabetes at 24–28 weeks (Chapter 10). Perineal culture for GBS carrier status at 35–36 weeks gestation (Chapter 24).

Obstetric Clinical Algorithms: Management and Evidence. By © E.R. Norwitz, M. Belfort, G.R. Saade and H. Miller.
Published 2010 Blackwell Publishing.

3. Additional genetic screening tests in the high-risk group to be screened include: sickle cell disease (African ethnicity), β-thalassemia (Mediterranean women), and Tay–Sachs disease, Canavan disease, Niemann–Pick disease, Bloom syndrome, familial dysautonomia, Fanconi anemia, and Gaucher disease in couples of Eastern European (Ashkenazi) Jewish extraction.

4. Major chromosomal abnormalities include trisomy 21 (Down syndrome, with an overall risk of 1/800 livebirths but strongly associated with maternal age), trisomy 18 (Edwards syndrome, 1/3500), trisomy 13 (Patau syndrome, 1/5000), and sex chromosomal disorders such as 47,XXY (Klinefelter syndrome, 1/500) and 45,X (Turner syndrome, 1/2500 livebirths but accounts for around 25% of early miscarriage). Many of these chromosomal disorders are due to nondisjunction events. Genetic abnormalities are classified according to the mode of genetic transmission: (i) autosomal dominant in 70% of cases (Huntington chorea, neurofibromatosis, achondroplasia, Marfan syndrome); (ii) autosomal recessive in 20% (sickle cell disease, cystic fibrosis, Tay–Sachs disease, β-thalassemia); (iii) X-linked recessive in 5% (Duchenne muscular dystrophy, hemophilia); (iv) X-linked dominant in <1% (vitamin D-resistant rickets); and (v) multifactorial inheritance in 3–5% (neural tube defect, club feet, hydrocephaly, cleft lip, cardiac anomalies).

5. Advanced maternal age (AMA) refers to women ≥35 years at delivery (see Chapter 32). Such women account for 5–8% of deliveries and 20–30% of Down syndrome births.

6. Chorionic villous sampling (CVS) can be offered for karyotype analysis at 9–14 weeks. CVS involves sampling of placental tissue which can be used for DNA analysis, cytogenetic testing or enzyme assays. Advantages include earlier diagnosis. Disadvantages include potential for maternal cell contamination and sampling of cells destined to become placenta rather than fetus. CVS performed <9 weeks is associated with a threefold increase in limb reduction defects. After 15 weeks, ultrasound-guided amniocentesis can be performed and amniocytes isolated for karyotype analysis. The procedure-related pregnancy loss rate for both procedures is estimated at 1/400. Early amniocentesis (<15 weeks) is associated with increased pregnancy loss and is thus not recommended.

7. Nuchal translucency (NT) measurements at 11–14 weeks correlate with fetal aneuploidy. A measurement of >2.5 mm is seen in 2–6% of fetuses of which 50–70% will have a chromosomal anomaly. However, it is not a sensitive enough test to use on its own. First-trimester risk assessment screening incorporates NT and the two maternal serum analyte markers, pregnancy-associated plasma protein-A (PAPP-A) and β-subunit of human chorionic gonadotropin (β-hCG).

8. Second-trimester maternal serum analyte screening uses a panel of biochemical markers to adjust the maternal age-related risk for fetal aneuploidy. The standard quadruple panel test ("quad test") at 15–20 weeks uses four maternal serum markers (AFP, β-hCG, estriol, and inhibin A). The most important variable is gestational age, which accounts for the majority of false-positive results.

9. Congenital anomalies refer to structural defects present at birth. Major congenital anomalies (those incompatible with life or requiring major surgery) occur in 2–3% of livebirths, and 5% of livebirths have minor malformations. Thirty to 40% of congenital anomalies have a known cause, including chromosomal abnormalities (0.5%), single gene defects (1%), multifactorial disorders, and teratogenic exposures. However, 60–70% have no known cause.

10. Elevated levels of maternal serum α-fetoprotein (MS-AFP) at 15–20 weeks (defined variably as ≥2.0 or ≥2.5 multiples of the median (MoM)) are associated with open neural tube defect (NTD) in high- and low-risk populations. A detailed sonographic exam of the fetal spine and head (for hydrocephalus, "lemon sign" and "banana sign") is indicated. If the spine and head are normal, consider other causes of elevated MS-AFP, including wrong dates, maternal hepatitis, twins, IUFD, IUGR, placental abruption, abnormal placentation, and other fetal anomalies (anterior abdominal wall defects, renal defects).

11. Fetal echocardiogram at 20–22 weeks is indicated in women at risk of having a fetus with a cardiac defect, including couples with a personal or family history of congenital heart disease, women with pregestational diabetes, an abnormal four-chamber and/or outflow tract view of the fetal heart on routine second-trimester ultrasound, select medication exposure in pregnancy (lithium, paroxetine), low PAPP-A at 11–14 weeks' gestation, and all IVF conceptions.

51 Preterm Labor

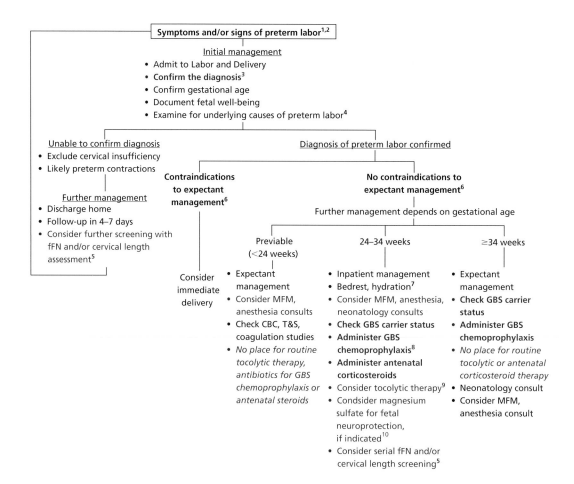

1. Labor is defined as an increase in myometrial activity resulting in effacement and dilation of the uterine cervix and delivery of the products of conception. Preterm labor refers to the onset of labor prior to 37 weeks of gestation. It occurs in 8–12% of deliveries, but accounts for >85% of perinatal mortality.

2. Several risk factors for preterm birth have been identified (see Chapter 52). However, >50% of spontaneous preterm births occur in women with no apparent risk factors. Moreover, although obstetric care providers are

getting better at identifying women at risk of preterm birth, it is not clear that this outcome can be prevented.

3. A definitive diagnosis of preterm labor is necessary before further treatment options are considered. Diagnosis requires the presence of both uterine contractions and cervical change (or, in nulliparous patients, an initial cervical exam >2 cm and/or >80% effacement in the setting of uterine contractions of increasing intensity and frequency). Uterine activity in the absence of cervical change should be regarded as preterm contractions, and does not require further treatment.

Obstetric Clinical Algorithms: Management and Evidence. By © E.R. Norwitz, M. Belfort, G.R. Saade and H. Miller.
Published 2010 Blackwell Publishing.

4. Preterm labor probably represents a syndrome rather than a diagnosis since the etiologies are varied. Of all preterm births, 20% are iatrogenic and performed for maternal or fetal indications, such as diabetes, placenta previa or IUGR. A further 20–30% result from intra-amniotic infection/inflammation, 20–25% occur in the setting of preterm PROM, and the remaining 25–30% are the result of spontaneous preterm labor.

5. Fetal fibronectin (fFN) testing and cervical length assessment are discussed further in Chapter 52.

6. Contraindications to expectant management include intrauterine infection, nonreassuring fetal testing ("fetal distress"), unexplained vaginal bleeding, and intrauterine fetal demise or a lethal fetal anomaly.

7. Bedrest and hydration are commonly recommended in the setting of preterm labor, but without proven efficacy.

8. Screening for GBS carrier status and GBS chemoprophylaxis are discussed further in Chapter 24.

9. Pharmacologic therapy remains the cornerstone of modern management of preterm labor. Although a number of alternative agents are now available (see table below), there are no reliable data to suggest that any of these agents is able to delay premature delivery for longer than a few days. No single agent has a clear therapeutic advantage; as such, the side-effect profile of each of the drugs will often determine which to use in a given clinical setting. The only agent approved by the FDA in the United States for the treatment of preterm labor is ritodrine hydrochloride (which is no longer on formulary in the US). Maintenance tocolytic therapy beyond 48 hours has not been shown to confer any therapeutic benefit, but does pose a significant risk of adverse side-effects. The concurrent use of two or more tocolytic agents has not been shown to be more effective than a single agent alone, and the additive risk of side-effects generally precludes this course of management. However, the use of sequential therapy (discontinuation of one agent followed by initiation of an alternative) may be beneficial.

10. Although controversial, recent data suggest that very low birthweight infants (<1500 g) exposed to iv magnesium suflate 12–24 hours prior to delivery may be partially protected against neurologic injury including cerebral palsy.

Common options for short-term tocolytic therapy			
Tocolytic agent	Route of administration (dosage)	Major maternal side-effects	Major fetal side-effects
Magnesium sulfate	IV (4–6 g bolus, then 2–3 g/h infusion)	Nausea, ileus, headache, weakness, hypotension, pulmonary edema, cardiorespiratory arrest	Decreased beat-to-beat variability, neonatal drowsiness, hypotonia, ?congenital ricketic syndrome
β-Adrenergic agonists Terbutaline sulfate	IV (2 μg/min infusion, max 80 μg/min) SC (0.25 mg q 20 min)	Jitteriness, anxiety, restlessness, nausea, vomiting, rash, cardiac dysrhythmias, myocardial ischemia, palpitations, chest pain, hypotension, tachycardia, pulmonary edema, paralytic ileus, hypokalemia, hyperglycemia, acidosis	Fetal tachycardia, hypotension, ileus, hyperinsulinemia, hypoglycemia, hyperbilirubinemia, hypocalcemia, ?hydrops fetalis
Prostaglandin inhibitors Indometacin	Oral (25–50 mg q 4–6 h) Rectal (100 mg q 12 h)	Gastrointestinal effects (nausea, heartburn), rash, headache, interstitial nephritis, ?increased bleeding time	Transient oliguria, oligohydramnios, ?necrotizing enterocolitis, ?intraventricular hemorrhage Premature closure of neonatal ductus arteriosus and persistent pulmonary hypertension
Calcium channel blockers Nifedipine	Oral (20–30 mg q 4–8 h)	Hypotension, reflex tachycardia, headache, nausea, flushing, potentiates the cardiac depressive effect of magnesium sulfate, hepatotoxicity	–

52 Screening for Preterm Birth

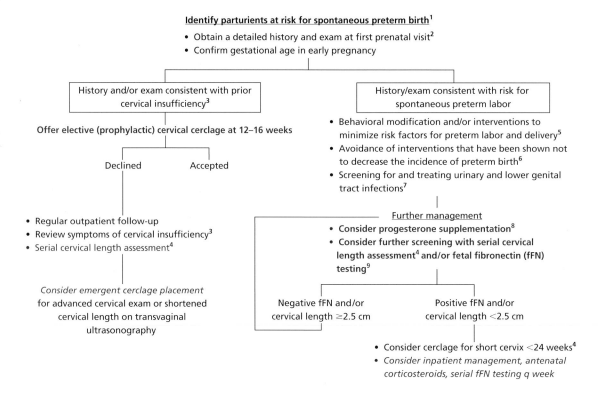

Identify parturients at risk for spontaneous preterm birth[1]
- Obtain a detailed history and exam at first prenatal visit[2]
- Confirm gestational age in early pregnancy

History and/or exam consistent with prior cervical insufficiency[3]

Offer elective (prophylactic) cervical cerclage at 12–16 weeks

Declined   Accepted

- Regular outpatient follow-up
- Review symptoms of cervical insufficiency[3]
- Serial cervical length assessment[4]

Consider emergent cerclage placement for advanced cervical exam or shortened cervical length on transvaginal ultrasonography

History/exam consistent with risk for spontaneous preterm labor

- Behavioral modification and/or interventions to minimize risk factors for preterm labor and delivery[5]
- Avoidance of interventions that have been shown not to decrease the incidence of preterm birth[6]
- Screening for and treating urinary and lower genital tract infections[7]

Further management
- **Consider progesterone supplementation[8]**
- **Consider further screening with serial cervical length assessment[4] and/or fetal fibronectin (fFN) testing[9]**

Negative fFN and/or cervical length ≥2.5 cm

Positive fFN and/or cervical length <2.5 cm

- Consider cerclage for short cervix <24 weeks[4]
- *Consider inpatient management, antenatal corticosteroids, serial fFN testing q week*

1. Twenty percent of preterm births are indication (iatrogenic) and performed for either maternal or fetal indications. A further 20–30% result from intra-amniotic infection/inflammation, 20–25% occur in the setting of preterm PROM (pPROM), and 25–30% are the result of spontaneous preterm labor. This algorithm deals only with the prevention of spontaneous preterm labor and delivery.

2. Risk factors associated with spontaneous preterm labor and delivery may be nonmodifiable or modifiable factors (see table below). In theory, identification of risk factors for preterm delivery before conception or early in pregnancy will facilitate interventions that may help prevent this complication. However, causality is difficult to assess and most preterm births occur among women with no risk factors. Furthermore, the number of effective interventions is limited.

3. See Chapter 35.

4. The relative risk of preterm birth increases as cervical length decreases. However, routine use of cervical ultrasonography for prediction of preterm birth in asymptomatic women is not currently recommended due to lack of effective interventions and low specificity. Data regarding the use of cervical cerclage for asymptomatic women with a shortened cervix (<2.5 cm) are conflicting; as such, this procedure cannot be routinely recommended.

Obstetric Clinical Algorithms: Management and Evidence. By © E.R. Norwitz, M. Belfort, G.R. Saade and H. Miller.
Published 2010 Blackwell Publishing.

Risk factors for preterm birth

Nonmodifiable risk factors

- Prior preterm birth
- African-American race
- Maternal age <18 or >40 years
- Low pre-pregnancy weight
- Low socio-economic status
- Chronic hypertension
- Intra-amniotic infection
- Diethylstilbestrol (DES) exposure
- Cervical injury or anomaly
- Uterine anomaly or fibroid
- Premature cervical dilation (>2 cm) or effacement (>80%)
- Overdistended uterus (multiple pregnancy, polyhydramnios)
- Vaginal bleeding
- ? Excessive uterine activity

Modifiable risk factors

- Smoking (≥10 cigarettes per day)
- Illicit drug use (especially cocaine)
- Absent prenatal care
- Short interpregnancy intervals
- Anemia
- Bacteriuria/urinary tract infection
- Genital infection
- ? Strenuous work during pregnancy
- ? High personal stress

5. Interventions that will likely decrease the risk of spontaneous preterm birth include smoking cessation, avoidance of illicit substance use (especially cocaine), avoidance of multiple pregnancies at ART, reduced occupational fatigue, and treatment of symptomatic genital infections. Interventions that may be recommended but are less likely to have a beneficial effect include an improvement in overall maternal nutrition (although there are no specific nutritional supplements which have been shown to decrease preterm birth) and regular antenatal care.

6. Several interventions have been shown in well-designed studies not to decrease the incidence of preterm birth and, as such, cannot routinely be recommended. These include home uterine activity monitoring, bedrest, broad-spectrum antibiotic therapy (in the absence of pPROM), and maintenance tocolytic therapy (such as long-term outpatient oral or intravenous β-agonist therapy; see Chapter 51).

7. All parturients should have a first-trimester urine culture to exclude asymptomatic bacteriuria. Regular antenatal screening is also recommended for women at risk for asymptomatic bacteriuria, including women with sickle cell trait, recurrent urinary tract infections, diabetes, and renal disease. Lower genital tract infections (such as BV, gonorrhea, chlamydia, ureaplasma, and trichomoniasis) have been associated with preterm birth. Symptomatic infections should be treated. Screening for chlamydia is recommended for all pregnant women, while screening for gonorrhea is recommended only for women at high risk. Routine screening of asymptomatic women for other lower genital tract infections cannot be recommended at this time.

8. Progesterone supplementation (17α-hydroxyprogesterone caproate) from 16–20 weeks through 34–36 weeks may reduce the rate of preterm birth in high-risk women. Further investigations are needed to evaluate the effectiveness of progesterone supplementation for decreasing the incidence of preterm delivery in high- and low-risk populations and to better understand its mechanism of action.

9. The fetal fibronectin (fFN) assay is likely the best predictor of preterm birth because of the low prevalence of positive results in asymptomatic low-risk women. However, sensitivity and positive predictive value are also low. Disadvantages are its cost and the need to collect cervicovaginal secretions from the posterior fornix using a speculum. According to ACOG, candidates for fFN testing include *symptomatic* women between 24–0/7 and 34–6/7 weeks of gestation with intact amniotic membranes and cervical dilation <3 cm. Under these conditions, 80% of women will be fFN negative (<50 ng/mL). A negative fFN effectively excludes imminent preterm delivery: <1% (1 in 125) of women will deliver within 14 days. A positive fFN test will predict delivery within the next 14 days in only 16% (1 in 6) of symptomatic women. As such, the value of the fFN test lies primarily in its negative predictive value (124 of 125 symptomatic women with a negative fFN test will not deliver within 14 days). If the fFN test is negative and clinical concern persists, consider repeating the test in 1–2 weeks.

53 Preterm Premature Rupture of the Membranes[1]

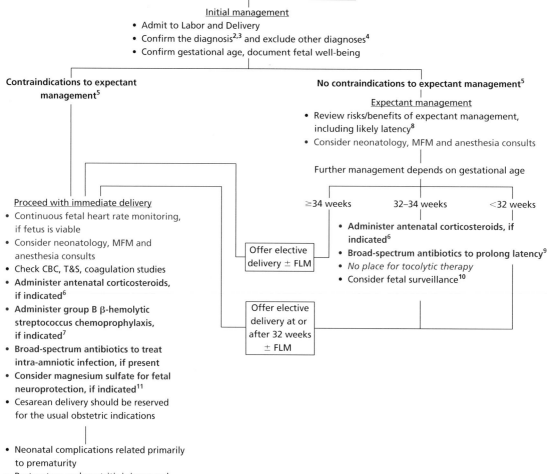

Symptoms and/or signs suggestive of pPROM[2]

Initial management
- Admit to Labor and Delivery
- Confirm the diagnosis[2,3] and exclude other diagnoses[4]
- Confirm gestational age, document fetal well-being

Contraindications to expectant management[5]

No contraindications to expectant management[5]

Expectant management
- Review risks/benefits of expectant management, including likely latency[8]
- Consider neonatology, MFM and anesthesia consults

Further management depends on gestational age

≥34 weeks   32–34 weeks   <32 weeks

Proceed with immediate delivery
- Continuous fetal heart rate monitoring, if fetus is viable
- Consider neonatology, MFM and anesthesia consults
- Check CBC, T&S, coagulation studies
- **Administer antenatal corticosteroids, if indicated[6]**
- **Administer group B β-hemolytic streptococcus chemoprophylaxis, if indicated[7]**
- **Broad-spectrum antibiotics to treat intra-amniotic infection, if present**
- **Consider magnesium sulfate for fetal neuroprotection, if indicated[11]**
- **Cesarean delivery should be reserved for the usual obstetric indications**

Offer elective delivery ± FLM

- **Administer antenatal corticosteroids, if indicated[6]**
- **Broad-spectrum antibiotics to prolong latency[9]**
- *No place for tocolytic therapy*
- **Consider fetal surveillance[10]**

Offer elective delivery at or after 32 weeks ± FLM

- Neonatal complications related primarily to prematurity
- Postpartum endometritis is increased after pPROM

1. Premature rupture of the membranes (PROM) refers to rupture of the fetal membranes prior to the onset of labor. It can occur at term or preterm. Preterm PROM (pPROM) refers to PROM prior to 37 weeks of gestation. This should not be confused with prolonged PROM, which refers to PROM for ≥24 hours and is associated with an increased risk of intra-amniotic infection. pPROM complicates 2–4% of all singleton and 7–10% of twin pregnancies. It is associated with 30–40% of preterm births, and 10% of all perinatal mortality. Risk factors for pPROM include prior pPROM (recurrence risk is 20–30% as compared with 4% in women with a prior uncomplicated delivery), placental abruption

Obstetric Clinical Algorithms: Management and Evidence. By © E.R. Norwitz, M. Belfort, G.R. Saade and H. Miller.
Published 2010 Blackwell Publishing.

(may account for 10–15% of pPROM), vaginal bleeding in the first or second trimester, cervical insufficiency, cervicovaginal infection or chorioamnionitis, amniocentesis, cigarette smoking, multiple gestation, polyhydramnios, chronic steroid treatment, *in utero* diethylstilbestrol (DES) exposure, connective tissue diseases (Ehlers–Danlos syndrome, SLE), anemia, low socio-economic status, and single women. Factors which are <u>not</u> associated with pPROM include coitus, cervical examinations, maternal exercise, and parity.

2. Preterm PROM is largely a <u>clinical</u> diagnosis. It is usually suggested by a history of watery vaginal discharge, and confirmed on sterile speculum examination by finding a pool of vaginal fluid which has an alkaline pH (it turns yellow nitrazine paper blue) and demonstrates microscopic ferning on drying. Findings of diminished amniotic fluid volume (by Leopold's exam or on ultrasound) may further suggest the diagnosis.

3. If the diagnosis is equivocal, transabdominal instillation of dye into the amniotic cavity (indigo carmine rather than methylene blue because of the association of methylene blue with methemoglobinemia) and documentation of leakage of dye into the vagina (by staining of a tampon within 20–30 min) will confirm the diagnosis. However, this amnio/dye test (or "tampon test") is rarely performed because of the risks of amniocentesis, which include PROM.

4. Differential diagnosis of PROM includes urinary incontinence, excessive vaginal discharge, and cervical mucus ("show").

5. The management of pPROM involves weighing the risk of prematurity against the risk of expectant management. Absolute contraindications to expectant management include intra-amniotic infection (chorioamnionitis), nonreassuring fetal testing or active labor. A favorable gestational age (likely ≥36 weeks) can be regarded as a relative contraindication to expectant management.

6. Administration of antenatal glucocorticoids has been shown to decrease the incidence of respiratory distress syndrome, intraventricular hemorrhage, and necrotizing enterocolitis if administered to pregnancies threatening to deliver prior to 34 weeks of gestation with intact membranes. A similar effect has been demonstrated in pregnancies complicated by pPROM prior to 32 weeks.

However, there is insufficient evidence to demonstrate a similar response to pregnancies complicated by pPROM from 32 to 34 weeks. There is no proven benefit to antenatal corticosteroids after 34 weeks. Multiple courses of steroids are not recommended. However, a repeat (salvage) course should be considered if the initial course was given prior to 28–32 weeks.

7. Intrapartum (not antepartum) group B β-hemolytic streptococcus chemoprophylaxis is indicated for all women with preterm labor, unless a negative perineal culture for group B β-hemolytic streptococcus has been documented within the prior 5 weeks. Intravenous penicillin is the antibiotic of choice.

8. Latency refers to the interval between rupture of the membranes and the onset of labor. In general, 50% of pregnancies complicated by pPROM will go into labor within 24–48 hours and 70–90% within 7 days. A number of factors affect latency including gestational age, oligohydramnios (severe oligohydramnios is associated with shortened latency), and multiple pregnancy (twins have a shorter latency period than singletons).

9. Prophylactic broad-spectrum antibiotics have been shown to prolong latency in the setting of pPROM. There is currently no evidence to recommend one regimen over another. The most common regimen is Ampicillin 2 g/erythromycin 250 mg IV q6h × 48 h followed by amoxicillin 250 mg/erythro 333 mg po q8h × 5 days.

10. Fetuses in pregnancies complicated by pPROM are at risk for infection, cord accident, placental abruption, and (possibly) uteroplacental insufficiency. While it is generally accepted that some form of fetal monitoring is necessary, the type and frequency of this monitoring are controversial. Options include weekly or daily nonstress testing and/or biophysical profile, but none has been shown to be superior to fetal kickcharts. Indeed, complications such as placental abruption, cord accident, and intra-amniotic infection cannot be predicted or reliably detected by such antenatal fetal testing.

11. Although controversial, recent data suggest that very low birthweight infants (<1500 g) exposed to iv magnesium sulfate 12–24 hours prior to delivery may be partially protected against neurologic injury including cerebral palsy.

54 Vaginal Birth after Cesarean

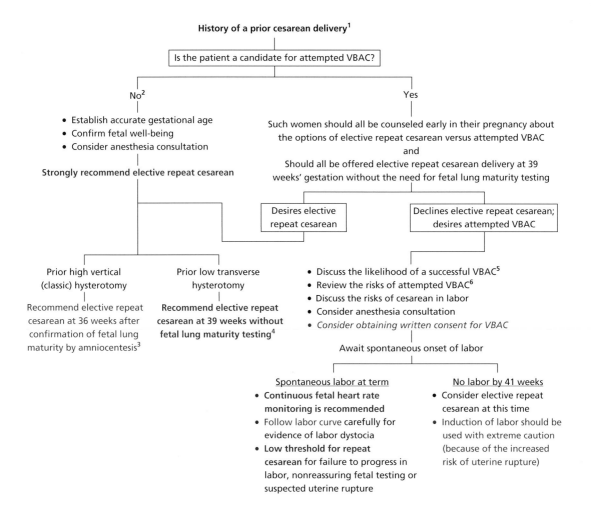

History of a prior cesarean delivery[1]

Is the patient a candidate for attempted VBAC?

No[2]

- Establish accurate gestational age
- Confirm fetal well-being
- Consider anesthesia consultation

Strongly recommend elective repeat cesarean

Yes

Such women should all be counseled early in their pregnancy about the options of elective repeat cesarean versus attempted VBAC

and

Should all be offered elective repeat cesarean delivery at 39 weeks' gestation without the need for fetal lung maturity testing

Desires elective repeat cesarean

Declines elective repeat cesarean; desires attempted VBAC

Prior high vertical (classic) hysterotomy

Recommend elective repeat cesarean at 36 weeks after confirmation of fetal lung maturity by amniocentesis[3]

Prior low transverse hysterotomy

Recommend elective repeat cesarean at 39 weeks without fetal lung maturity testing[4]

- Discuss the likelihood of a successful VBAC[5]
- Review the risks of attempted VBAC[6]
- Discuss the risks of cesarean in labor
- Consider anesthesia consultation
- *Consider obtaining written consent for VBAC*

Await spontaneous onset of labor

<u>Spontaneous labor at term</u>
- **Continuous fetal heart rate monitoring is recommended**
- Follow labor curve **carefully for evidence of labor dystocia**
- **Low threshold for repeat cesarean** for failure to progress in labor, nonreassuring fetal testing or suspected uterine rupture

<u>No labor by 41 weeks</u>
- Consider elective repeat cesarean at this time
- Induction of labor should be used with extreme caution (because of the increased risk of uterine rupture)

Obstetric Clinical Algorithms: Management and Evidence. By © E.R. Norwitz, M. Belfort, G.R. Saade and H. Miller.
Published 2010 Blackwell Publishing.

1. Cesarean delivery refers to delivery of a fetus via the abdominal route (laparotomy) requiring an incision into the uterus (hysterotomy). It is now the second most common surgical procedure (behind male circumcision), accounting for around 20–25% of all deliveries in the UK and 30% of deliveries in the US. Approximately one-third of cesarean deliveries are elective repeat procedures.

2. *Absolute contraindications* for attempted VBAC include one or more prior high vertical ("classic") cesarean deliveries, nonreassuring fetal testing ("fetal distress"), transverse lie, placenta previa or delivery in a setting that is unable to supply immediate access to anesthesia services or unable to perform an emergency cesarean. *Relative contraindications* include more than one prior cesarean, breech presentation, prior full-thickness myomectomy or a prior uterine rupture.

3. In women who have had one or more prior high vertical ("classic") cesarean deliveries, an elective repeat cesarean should be performed at 36 weeks' gestation prior to the onset of labor and after confirmation of fetal lung maturity by amniocentesis. This is because of the high risk of uterine rupture in such women (4–8%) and the knowledge that 50% of such uterine ruptures occur prior to labor.

4. According to the ACOG, elective repeat cesarean can be performed after 39–0/7 weeks in a well-dated pregnancy without documenting fetal lung maturity by amniocentesis. In HIV-positive women and twins, an elective cesarean without amniocentesis can be performed after 38–0/7 weeks.

5. A successful VBAC can be achieved in 65–80% of women. Factors associated with successful VBAC include one or more prior vaginal deliveries, estimated fetal weight <4000 g, and a nonrecurrent indication for the prior cesarean (breech, placenta previa) rather than a potentially recurrent indication (such as cephalopelvic disproportion).

6. Attempted VBAC is associated with a number of risks.
- Failed VBAC leading to <u>emergency cesarean delivery</u> with a associated increased risk of maternal mortality (approximately 0.01%; 2–10-fold higher than for vaginal birth and elective cesarean prior to labor) and morbidity (infection, thromboembolic events, wound dehiscence).
- <u>Uterine rupture,</u> which may be life-threatening. Symptoms and signs of uterine rupture include acute onset of fetal bradycardia (70%), abdominal pain (10%), vaginal bleeding (5%), hemodynamic instability (5–10%), and/or loss of the presenting part (<5%). Epidural anesthesia may mask some of these features. Risk factors for uterine rupture include the type of prior uterine incision (<1% for lower segment transverse incision, 2–3% for lower segment vertical, and 4–8% for high vertical), two or more prior cesareans (4%), prior uterine rupture, "excessive" use of oxytocin (although the term "excessive" is poorly defined), dysfunctional labor pattern (especially prolonged second stage or arrest of dilation), and induction of labor (especially with the use of prostaglandins). Factors not associated with uterine rupture include epidural anesthesia, unknown uterine scar, fetal macrosomia, and indication for prior cesarean. Uterine rupture is associated with significant maternal mortality and morbidity (including the need for emergency cesarean and possible blood transfusion) as well as a fivefold increased risk of fetal morbidity (hypoxic ischemic brain injury) and death. NOTE: Uterine rupture should be distinguished from uterine dehiscence, which refers to subclinical separation of the prior uterine incision that is often detected only by manual exploration of the scar following vaginal delivery or at the time of elective cesarean. It occurs in 2–3% of women with a prior cesarean delivery. In the absence of vaginal bleeding, no further treatment is necessary.
- Increased risk of *puerperal (cesarean) hysterectomy*. This is a rare event (1 in 6000 deliveries) that is performed primarily as an emergency when the mother's life is at risk due to uncontrolled hemorrhage. It is a highly morbid procedure and is therefore performed only as a last resort. Warming blanket, three-way Foley catheter, and blood products should be available. Blood loss is often excessive (2–4 L) and blood transfusions are usually required (90%). Despite a high morbidity, overall maternal mortality is low (0.3%). Although women will subsequently be amenorrheic and sterile, menopausal symptoms will not develop if the ovaries are left.

55 Teratology[1]

- Take a detailed history and perform a physical examination. Ask specifically about exposure to medications, illicit and social drug use, infections, and environmental toxins
- Understand changes in pharmacokinetics/pharmacodynamics during pregnancy and how these alter drug levels and efficacy[2]
- Be aware of the FDA classification of drugs in pregnancy[3]

Medications[4]

Not considered teratogenic	Proven teratogens in humans	
• Folic acid	• Androgens	• Phenytoin
• Synthroid	(→ virilization)	(→ CNS defects, IUGR)
• Anesthetic agents	• ACE inhibitors	• Streptomycin
• Acetaminophen	(→ renal damage)	(→ deafness)
• Aspirin	• Antithyroid drugs	• Warfarin
• Antiemetics/	(→ thyroid injury)	(→ embryopathy, IUGR)
antihistamines	• Carbamazepine	• Tetracyline
• Acyclovir	(→ NTD, IUGR)	(→ bone/teeth defects)
• Heparin	• Cyclophosphamide	• Thalidomide
• Metronidazole	(→ CNS defects)	(→ limb/ear defects)
• Iron supplementation	• Folate antagonists	• Valproic acid
• Oral contraceptives	(→ CNS defects)	(→ NTD)
• Trimethoprim	• Lithium	• Vitamin A
• Zidovudine (AZT)	(→ cardiac defects)	(→ CNS defects)

Environmental toxins[5]

- Illicit drugs (cocaine, marijuana)[6]
- Social drugs (alcohol, nicotine, caffeine)[7]
- Radiation exposure
- Heat
- ? Electromagnetic field exposure

Antepartum considerations
- **Only use medications in pregnancy if absolutely indicated**
- **If possible, avoid initiating therapy in the first trimester**
- Select a safe medication (preferably an older drug with a proven track record in pregnancy)
- **Use the lowest effective dose**
- **Single-agent therapy is preferable**
- *Discourage the use of over-the-counter drugs*

- **Sonographic fetal anatomic survey at 18–22 weeks**
- Consider MFM consultation
- Adjust medications with approval of appropriate consultations

1. Teratology refers to the study of abnormal fetal development, and includes both structural and functional abnormalities.

2. Pharmacokinetics is the study of how a drug moves through the body. Drug absorption is altered in pregnancy because gastric emptying and intestinal motility are decreased. Pulmonary tidal volume is increased which affects absorption of inhaled drugs. The volume of distribution changes in pregnancy, with a 40% increase in plasma volume, 7–8 L increase in total body water, and 20–40% increase in body fat. Despite these changes (which decrease drug levels), albumin declines and free fatty acid and lipoprotein levels rise. As a result, protein binding of many drugs is decreased in pregnancy, leading to an increase in circulating free (biologically active) drug levels. Drug metabolism and elimination also change in

Obstetric Clinical Algorithms: Management and Evidence. By © E.R. Norwitz, M. Belfort, G.R. Saade and H. Miller.
Published 2010 Blackwell Publishing.

pregnancy. High steroid hormone levels affect hepatic metabolism and prolong the half-life of some drugs. Glomerular filtration rate rise by 50–60%, thereby increasing the renal clearance of other drugs.

3. The FDA has defined five risk categories for drug use in pregnancy (see table below). Individual agents are assigned to a risk category according to their risk/benefit ratio (e.g. oral contraceptives are not teratogenic, but are classified as category X because there is no benefit to being on the pill once you are pregnant).

4. Twenty to 25% of women report using medications on a regular basis throughout pregnancy. Major conge-nital anomalies occur in 3–4% of livebirths, and 70% of such anomalies have no known cause. It is estimated that 2–3% are due to medications and 1% to environmental toxins. With the exception of large molecules (such as heparin), all drugs given to the mother cross the placenta to some degree. The effect of a given drug on a fetus depends on dose, time and duration of exposure as well as poorly defined genetic and environmental factors. A fetus is at highest risk for injury during embryogenesis (days 17–54 postconception). Paternal exposure has never been shown to be teratogenic. Drug trials are difficult to carry out in pregnancy because of concern over the fetus. As such, many drugs have not been validated for use or safety in human pregnancy. Recommendations often rely on data from animal models. The occurrence of thalidomide-associated embryopathy has led to the belief that human teratogenicity cannot be predicted by animal studies. However, every drug that has since been found to be teratogenic in humans has caused similar effects in animals.

5. A number of environmental toxins have been implicated in fetal injury: (i) ionizing radiation has been associated with spontaneous abortion, microcephaly, mental retardation, and (possibly) malignancy in later life. Fetal exposure of at least >5 Rad is required for any adverse effect, which is 1000-fold higher than most imaging studies (estimated fetal exposure from common radiologic procedures is 1–3 mRad); (ii) heat has been weakly associated with spontaneous abortion and neural tube defects; (iii) electromagnetic field exposure has not consistently been shown to be injurious to the fetus.

6. The illicit drug which has been most commonly implicated in fetal injury is cocaine, which has been associated with IUGR, cerebral infarction, and placental abruption. Reported congenital anomalies (limb reduction defects, porencephalic cysts, microcephaly, bowel atresia, necrotizing enterocolitis, and long-term behavioral effects) may be secondary to cocaine-induced vasospasm. Marijuana has no clear teratogenic effects, but a weak and inconsistent association between marijuana and preterm birth, IUGR, and neurodevelopmental delay has been proposed.

7. A number of social drugs have been implicated in fetal injury. (i) Alcohol causes fetal alcohol syndrome, which is characterized by facial abnormalities (midfacial hypoplasia), central nervous system dysfunction (microcephaly, mental retardation), and IUGR. Renal and cardiac defects may also occur. The risk of anomalies is related to the extent of alcohol use: 10% with rare use, 15% with moderate use, and 30–40% with heavy use (>6 drinks per day). There is no safe level of alcohol use in pregnancy. (ii) Cigarette smoking is associated with subfertility, spontaneous abortion, preterm birth, perinatal mortality, and low-birthweight infants. Neonatal exposure is associated with SIDS, asthma, respiratory infections, and attention deficit disorder. Twenty to 30% of women continue to smoke during pregnancy. (iii) Caffeine has no clear teratogenic effects, but has been weakly associated with spontaneous abortion.

The FDA classification of drugs in pregnancy

Category	Criteria	Examples
A	Well-controlled studies in pregnant women have not shown an increased risk of fetal abnormalities	Vitamin C, folic acid, L-thyroxine
B	Animal studies have shown no evidence of harm to the fetus or have confirmed an adverse effect in the fetus, but there are no adequate and well-controlled studies in pregnant women	Benadryl, xylocaine, α-methyldopa, ampicillin, hydrochlorothiazide
C	There are no adequate or well-controlled studies in pregnant women	Theophylline, nifedipine, β-blockers, digoxin, acyclovir, zidovudine (AZT)
D	Studies in pregnant women have demonstrated a risk to the fetus. However, the benefits of therapy may outweigh the potential risk	Cytoxan, ACE inhibitors, phenytoin, spironolactone, methotrexate
X	Studies in animals or pregnant women have shown evidence of fetal abnormalities. The use of the product is contraindicated in women who are or may become pregnant	Radioisotopes, isotretinoin (vitamin A), oral contraceptives

56 Term Premature Rupture of the Membranes[1]

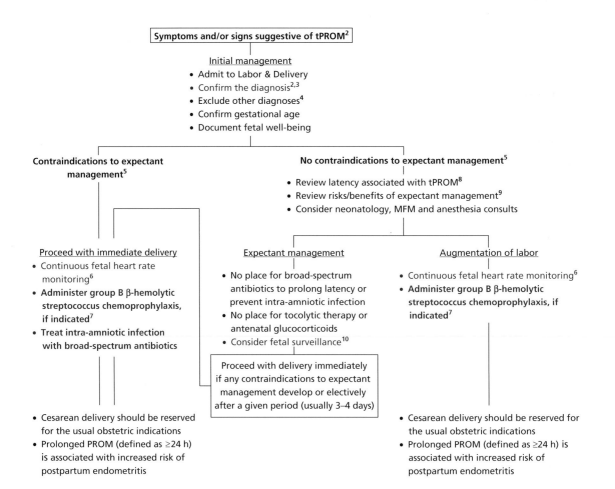

Symptoms and/or signs suggestive of tPROM[2]

Initial management
- Admit to Labor & Delivery
- Confirm the diagnosis[2,3]
- Exclude other diagnoses[4]
- Confirm gestational age
- Document fetal well-being

Contraindications to expectant management[5]

No contraindications to expectant management[5]
- Review latency associated with tPROM[8]
- Review risks/benefits of expectant management[9]
- Consider neonatology, MFM and anesthesia consults

Proceed with immediate delivery
- Continuous fetal heart rate monitoring[6]
- **Administer group B β-hemolytic streptococcus chemoprophylaxis, if indicated[7]**
- **Treat intra-amniotic infection with broad-spectrum antibiotics**

Expectant management
- No place for broad-spectrum antibiotics to prolong latency or prevent intra-amniotic infection
- No place for tocolytic therapy or antenatal glucocorticoids
- Consider fetal surveillance[10]

Proceed with delivery immediately if any contraindications to expectant management develop or electively after a given period (usually 3–4 days)

Augmentation of labor
- Continuous fetal heart rate monitoring[6]
- **Administer group B β-hemolytic streptococcus chemoprophylaxis, if indicated[7]**

- Cesarean delivery should be reserved for the usual obstetric indications
- Prolonged PROM (defined as ≥24 h) is associated with increased risk of postpartum endometritis

- Cesarean delivery should be reserved for the usual obstetric indications
- Prolonged PROM (defined as ≥24 h) is associated with increased risk of postpartum endometritis

Obstetric Clinical Algorithms: Management and Evidence. By © E.R. Norwitz, M. Belfort, G.R. Saade and H. Miller.
Published 2010 Blackwell Publishing.

1. Premature rupture of the membranes (PROM) refers to rupture of the fetal membranes prior to the onset of labor. It can occur at term or preterm. Term PROM (tPROM) refers to PROM occurring at or after 37 weeks of gestation. tPROM complicates 8–10% of all term pregnancies.

2. Term PROM is largely a clinical diagnosis. It is usually suggested by a history of watery vaginal discharge and confirmed on sterile speculum examination by finding a pool of vaginal fluid which has an alkaline pH (it turns yellow nitrazine paper blue) and demonstrates microscopic ferning on drying. Findings of diminished amniotic fluid volume (by Leopold's exam or on ultrasound) may further suggest the diagnosis.

3. Although used to confirm the diagnosis of preterm PROM remote from term, there is no place for the amnio/dye test (transabdominal instillation of dye into the amniotic cavity and documentation of leakage of dye into the vagina by staining of a tampon within 20–30 min; "tampon test") to confirm the diagnosis.

4. Differential diagnosis of tPROM includes urinary incontinence, excessive vaginal discharge, and cervical mucus ("show").

5. Contraindications to expectant management include intra-amniotic infection (chorioamnionitis), nonreassuring fetal testing, unexplained vaginal bleeding or labor.

6. Severe oligohydramnios results in an increased incidence of cord compression and nonreassuring fetal testing in labor leading to cesarean delivery. In this setting, amnioinfusion has been shown to improve fetal testing and decrease the cesarean delivery rate.

7. Intrapartum (not antepartum) group B β-hemolytic streptococcus (GBS) chemoprophylaxis is indicated for all women who have been identified as being GBS carriers by routine perineal culture at 35–36 weeks of gestation. If the patient's GBS carrier status is unknown, she should be given chemoprophylaxis if any risk factors are present (including premature labor, GBS bacteriuria during pregnancy, prolonged rupture of membranes defined as ≥18 hours, fever in labor, or prior GBS-infected infant). Intravenous penicillin is the antibiotic of choice.

8. Latency refers to the interval between rupture of the membranes and the onset of labor. In general, 50% of women with tPROM will go into labor spontaneously within 12 hours, 70% within 24 hours, 85% within 48 hours, and 95% within 72 hours. A number of factors affect latency including gestational age, oligohydramnios (severe oligohydramnios is associated with shortened latency), and multiple pregnancy (twins have a shorter latency period than singletons).

9. In the absence of any contraindications to delaying delivery, both expectant management and immediate augmentation of labor are acceptable. Patient management should therefore be individualized. If the cervix is unfavorable (effacement <80%, dilation <2 cm) and the patient is nulliparous, augmentation of labor may be associated with an increased incidence of cesarean delivery and intra-amniotic infection.

10. While it is generally accepted that some form of fetal monitoring is necessary, the type and frequency of this monitoring are controversial. Options include twice-weekly or daily nonstress testing and/or biophysical profile, but none has been shown to be superior to fetal kickcharts. Indeed, complications such as placental abruption, cord accident, and intra-amniotic infection cannot be predicted or reliably detected by such antenatal fetal testing.

57 Twin Pregnancy

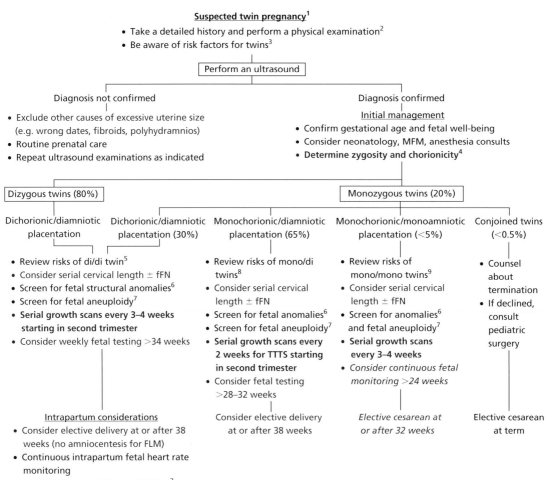

Suspected twin pregnancy[1]
- Take a detailed history and perform a physical examination[2]
- Be aware of risk factors for twins[3]

Perform an ultrasound

Diagnosis not confirmed
- Exclude other causes of excessive uterine size (e.g. wrong dates, fibroids, polyhydramnios)
- Routine prenatal care
- Repeat ultrasound examinations as indicated

Diagnosis confirmed

Initial management
- Confirm gestational age and fetal well-being
- Consider neonatology, MFM, anesthesia consults
- **Determine zygosity and chorionicity[4]**

Dizygous twins (80%)

Monozygous twins (20%)

Dichorionic/diamniotic placentation
- Review risks of di/di twin[5]
- Consider serial cervical length ± fFN
- Screen for fetal structural anomalies[6]
- Screen for fetal aneuploidy[7]
- **Serial growth scans every 3–4 weeks starting in second trimester**
- Consider weekly fetal testing >34 weeks

Dichorionic/diamniotic placentation (30%)

Monochorionic/diamniotic placentation (65%)
- Review risks of mono/di twins[8]
- Consider serial cervical length ± fFN
- Screen for fetal anomalies[6]
- Screen for fetal aneuploidy[7]
- **Serial growth scans every 2 weeks for TTTS starting in second trimester**
- Consider fetal testing >28–32 weeks

Consider elective delivery at or after 38 weeks

Monochorionic/monoamniotic placentation (<5%)
- Review risks of mono/mono twins[9]
- Consider serial cervical length ± fFN
- Screen for anomalies[6] and fetal aneuploidy[7]
- **Serial growth scans every 3–4 weeks**
- *Consider continuous fetal monitoring >24 weeks*

Elective cesarean at or after 32 weeks

Conjoined twins (<0.5%)
- Counsel about termination
- If declined, consult pediatric surgery

Elective cesarean at term

Intrapartum considerations
- Consider elective delivery at or after 38 weeks (no amniocentesis for FLM)
- Continuous intrapartum fetal heart rate monitoring
- Document presentation and EFW ×2
- Review mode of delivery[10]

Obstetric Clinical Algorithms: Management and Evidence. By © E.R. Norwitz, M. Belfort, G.R. Saade and H. Miller. Published 2010 Blackwell Publishing.

1. Multiple pregnancies complicate 1–2% of all deliveries and are becoming increasingly common, primarily as a result of assisted reproductive technology (ART). The vast majority (97–98%) of multiple gestations are twin pregnancies.

2. Suspect twins in women with excessive symptoms of pregnancy (e.g. nausea and vomiting) or uterine size larger than expected for gestational age.

3. Risk factors for twins include a family or personal history of dizygous twins (derived from two separate embryos), advanced maternal age, multiparity, African-American race, and ART. A history of monozygous twins is not a risk factor since it is a random event that occurs in 1 in 300 pregnancies.

4. Ultrasound will confirm the diagnosis, gestational age, fetal well-being, and chorionicity. Chorionicity refers to the arrangement of the fetal membranes. All dizygous twins have dichorionic/diamniotic placentation. In monozygous twins, the timing of the cell division determines the chorionicity. If the zygote divides within 3 days of fertilization, the result is dichorionic/diamniotic placentation; if the division occurs on days 3–8, the result is monochorionic/diamniotic placentation; days 8–13, monochorionic/monoamniotic placentation; and after day 13, incomplete separation (conjoined twins). Chorionicity correlates directly with perinatal mortality. Ultrasound examination in early pregnancy can determine if the placentation is dichorionic ("twin peak" or lambda sign) or monochorionic (no peak and a thin filmy membrane). Identification of separate-sex fetuses or two separate placentae confirms di/di placentation. Chorionicity is determined most accurately by examination of the membranes after delivery.

5. Antepartum complications develop in 80% of twins versus 20–30% of singleton pregnancies. Preterm birth is the most common complication. Fetal growth discordance (defined as ≥25% difference in EFW) occurs in 5–15% of twins, and is associated with a sixfold increase in perinatal mortality. Maternal complications include an increased risk of gestational diabetes, pre-eclampsia, preterm premature rupture of membranes, anemia, cholestasis of pregnancy, cesarean delivery (due primarily to malpresentation), and postpartum hemorrhage. Other fetal complications include an increased risk of fetal structural anomalies, IUFD of one or both twins (see Chapter 39), twin-to-twin transfusion syndrome (TTTS), twin reverse arterial perfusion (TRAP) sequence, and cord entanglement.

6. Twins are at increased risk of fetal structural anomalies compared with singletons. A detailed fetal anatomic survey of both fetuses is indicated at 18–20 weeks. Fetal echocardiography is not routinely recommended in twins.

7. Maternal serum α-fetoprotein (MS-AFP) and "quadruple panel" screening (MS-AFP, estriol, hCG, and inhibin A) have been standardized for twins as they are for singletons at 15–20 weeks. First-trimester risk assessment (nuchal translucency + serum PAPP-A and β-hCG) at 11–14 weeks is rapidly becoming the preferred aneuploidy screening test for multiple pregnancies. In dizygous pregnancies, the risk of aneuploidy is independent for each fetus. As such, the chance that one or both fetuses have a karyotypic abnormality is greater than for a singleton. Amniocentesis is typically recommended when the probability of aneuploidy is equal to or greater than the procedure-related pregnancy loss rate (estimated at 1 in 400).

8. Di/di twins do not share a blood supply. On the other hand, vascular communications can be demonstrated in almost 100% of mono/di twins. TTTS results from an imbalance in blood flow from the "donor" twin to the "recipient" and is seen in 15% of mono/di twin pregnancies. Both twins are at risk for adverse events. Following delivery, a difference in birthweight of ≥20% or a difference in hematocrit of ≥5 g/dL confirms the diagnosis. Prognosis depends on gestational age, severity, and underlying etiology. Overall perinatal mortality is 40–80%. Treatment options include expectant management, serial amniocentesis of the polyhydramniotic sac, indomethacin (to decrease fetal urine output), laser obliteration of the placental vascular communications, or selective fetal reduction.

9. Perinatal mortality is high with mono/mono twins (65–70%), due primarily to cord entanglement. As such, delivery should be by cesarean.

10. Route of delivery of twins depends on gestational age, EFW, presentation, and maternal and fetal well-being (see Chapter 62).

SECTION 5

Intrapartum/Postpartum Complications

58 Breech Presentation

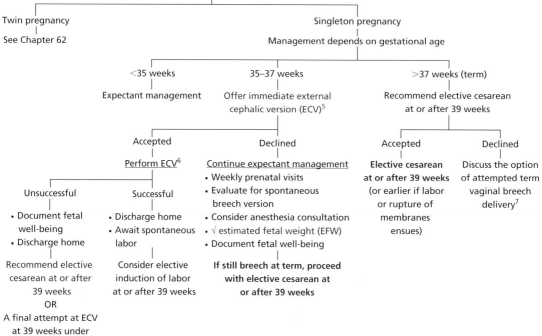

Suspect breech presentation[1]
- Take a detailed history, perform a physical examination, and perform relevant imaging tests[2]
- Recognize risk factors for breech presentation[3]
- Be aware of the risks associated with breech presentation[40]

Confirm breech presentation on ultrasound

Twin pregnancy

See Chapter 62

Singleton pregnancy

Management depends on gestational age

<35 weeks

Expectant management

35–37 weeks

Offer immediate external cephalic version (ECV)[5]

>37 weeks (term)

Recommend elective cesarean at or after 39 weeks

Accepted

Perform ECV[6]

Declined

Continue expectant management
- Weekly prenatal visits
- Evaluate for spontaneous breech version
- Consider anesthesia consultation
- √ estimated fetal weight (EFW)
- Document fetal well-being

If still breech at term, proceed with elective cesarean at or after 39 weeks

Accepted

Elective cesarean at or after 39 weeks (or earlier if labor or rupture of membranes ensues)

Declined

Discuss the option of attempted term vaginal breech delivery[7]

Unsuccessful
- Document fetal well-being
- Discharge home

Recommend elective cesarean at or after 39 weeks
OR
A final attempt at ECV at 39 weeks under epidural analgesia

Successful
- Discharge home
- Await spontaneous labor

Consider elective induction of labor at or after 39 weeks

Obstetric Clinical Algorithms: Management and Evidence. By © E.R. Norwitz, M. Belfort, G.R. Saade and H. Miller.
Published 2010 Blackwell Publishing.

1. Breech presentation refers to presentation of the fetal buttocks and/or lower extremities at the pelvic inlet. The incidence depends on gestational age: 30% at 28 weeks, 15% at 32 weeks, and 3–4% at term.

2. The diagnosis of breech presentation can be made by physical examination (Leopold's maneuvers), vaginal examination or ultrasound. Ultrasound will also determine the type of breech: frank (where legs are extended over the fetus's head – 70%), complete (where the legs are tucked into the so-called "fetal position" – 10%) or incomplete/footling breech (where a foot extends below the buttocks – 20%).

3. Risk factors for breech presentation include prematurity, uterine anomaly (such as uterine septum), polyhydramnios, prior term breech presentation, multiple pregnancy, placenta previa, and fetal anomalies (such as anencephaly or hydrocephalus).

4. Breech presentation is associated with a twofold increased risk of fetal structural anomalies. Such pregnancies are also at increased risk of adverse pregnancy outcome, including preterm labor, cord prolapse, birth trauma, and maternal morbidity (such as postpartum hemorrhage and severe perineal injury).

5. *External cephalic version* (ECV) refers to the attempted conversion of breech to vertex by manual manipulation through the maternal abdomen. It is best performed at 35–36 weeks' gestation. Contraindications to ECV may be absolute (placenta previa, nonreassuring fetal testing, preterm premature rupture of membranes or any contraindication to subsequent vaginal delivery such as a prior "classic" cesarean delivery) or relative (prior low transverse cesarean delivery, IUGR, twins, oligohydramnios or labor). ECV is associated with complications, including nonreassuring fetal testing ("fetal distress"), placental abruption, rupture of fetal membranes, need to emergent cesarean delivery, Rh isoimmunization, and (rarely) fetal neurologic injury or death.

6. Prior to performing ECV, the obstetric care provider should confirm breech presentation on ultrasound, document gestational age and fetal well-being (reactive NST), ensure that no contraindications are present (such as labor or ruptured membranes), and obtain written consent. Anti-Rh(D) immunoglobulin should be administered to prevent Rh isoimmunization, if indicated. ECV should be performed under ultrasound guidance. A short-acting tocolytic agent (such as the β-adrenergic agonist terbutaline) and/or epidural analgesia have been shown to improve the success rate of ECV, and can be used in selected cases. The overall success rate of ECV is 50–70%. Predictors of success include frank breech, normal or increased amniotic fluid volume, an experienced operator, a nonengaged breech, a multiparous and thin patient, and a laterally located fetal spine. An NST should be performed after ECV to document fetal well-being regardless of whether or not the ECV was successful.

7. Preterm singleton breech fetuses are best delivered by cesarean due, in large part, to the risk of entrapment of the aftercoming head. Management of the breech-presenting second twin is reviewed in Chapter 62. Although controversial, the weight of evidence suggests that singleton term breech fetuses are most safely delivered by cesarean, because of the attendant risks of vaginal breech delivery including cord prolapse, birth trauma, entrapment of the aftercoming head, birth asphyxia, and death. That said, vaginal breech delivery may be a safe alternative to elective cesarean under certain circumstances: (i) term frank breech; (ii) estimated fetal weight 2500–4000 g; (iii) no hyperextension ("star gazing") of the fetal head; (iv) immediate availability of emergency cesarean, if needed; (v) an experienced operator; (vi) adequate analgesia; (vii) confirmed fetal well-being; and (viii) ideally a woman who has had a prior successful vaginal delivery ("proven pelvis").

59 Intrapartum Fetal Testing[1]

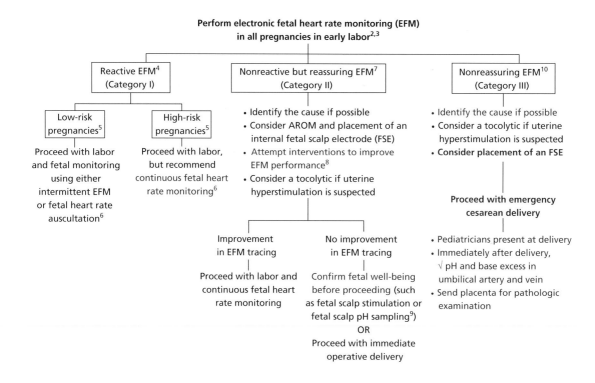

Perform electronic fetal heart rate monitoring (EFM)
in all pregnancies in early labor[2,3]

Reactive EFM[4]
(Category I)

Nonreactive but reassuring EFM[7]
(Category II)

Nonreassuring EFM[10]
(Category III)

Low-risk
pregnancies[5]

High-risk
pregnancies[5]

Proceed with labor
and fetal monitoring
using either
intermittent EFM
or fetal heart rate
auscultation[6]

Proceed with labor,
but recommend
continuous fetal heart
rate monitoring[6]

- Identify the cause if possible
- Consider AROM and placement of an
  internal fetal scalp electrode (FSE)
- Attempt interventions to improve
  EFM performance[8]
- Consider a tocolytic if uterine
  hyperstimulation is suspected

- Identify the cause if possible
- Consider a tocolytic if uterine
  hyperstimulation is suspected
- **Consider placement of an FSE**

**Proceed with emergency
cesarean delivery**

Improvement
in EFM tracing

No improvement
in EFM tracing

Proceed with labor and
continuous fetal heart
rate monitoring

Confirm fetal well-being
before proceeding (such
as fetal scalp stimulation or
fetal scalp pH sampling[9])
OR
Proceed with immediate
operative delivery

- Pediatricians present at delivery
- Immediately after delivery,
  √ pH and base excess in
  umbilical artery and vein
- Send placenta for pathologic
  examination

1. Fetal morbidity and mortality can occur as a consequence of labor. A number of tests have therefore been developed to assess fetal well-being in labor. Attention has focused on hypoxic ischemic encephalopathy (HIE) as a marker of birth asphyxia and a predictor of long-term outcome. HIE is a clinical condition that develops within the first hours or days of life. It is characterized by abnormalities of tone and feeding, alterations in consciousness, and convulsions. In order to attribute such a state to birth asphyxia, the following four criteria must all be fulfilled: (i) profound metabolic or mixed acidemia (pH <7.00) on an umbilical cord arterial blood sample, if obtained; (ii) Apgar score of 0–3 for longer than 5 min; (iii) neonatal neurologic manifestations (seizures,

coma); and (iv) multisystem organ dysfunction. At most, only 15% of cerebral palsy and mental retardation can be attributed to HIE.

2. Electronic fetal heart rate monitoring (EFM), also known as cardiotocography (CTG), refers to changes in the fetal heart rate pattern with time. It reflects maturity of the fetal autonomic nervous system. External EFM is noninvasive, simple to perform, readily available, and inexpensive. EFM interpretation is largely subjective and should always take into account gestational age, the presence or absence of congenital anomalies, and underlying clinical risk factors. Fetuses who are premature or growth restricted are less likely to tolerate episodes of decreased

Obstetric Clinical Algorithms: Management and Evidence. By © E.R. Norwitz, M. Belfort, G.R. Saade and H. Miller.
Published 2010 Blackwell Publishing.

placental perfusion and, as such, may be more prone to hypoxia and acidosis during labor. Drugs can also affect heart rate and variability.

3. Biophysical profile (BPP), umbilical artery Doppler velocimetry, and contraction stress test (CST) have not been well validated for use in labor. As such, they should not be used to document fetal well-being in labor.

4. A "reactive" EFM – defined as a normal baseline heart rate (110–160 bpm), moderate variability (which refers to peak-to-trough excursions of 5–25 bpm around the baseline), and at least two accelerations in 20 min each lasting ≥15 s and peaking at ≥15 bpm above baseline (or ≥10 bpm for ≥10 s if <32 weeks) – is reassuring and is associated with normal neurologic outcome. According to the 2008 NICHD Workshop Report on electronic fetal monitoring, this is referred to as a "Category I" tracing.

5. The designations "low-risk" and "high-risk" pregnancies refer to whether or not pregnancies are at risk of uteroplacental insufficiency (see Chapter 33).

6. When compared with intermittent fetal heart rate auscultation, continuous fetal heart rate monitoring during labor is associated with a decrease in the incidence of seizures in the first 28 days of life, but no difference in other measures of short-term perinatal morbidity or mortality. Moreover, the increase in neonatal seizures does not translate into differences in long-term morbidity (cerebral palsy, mental retardation or seizures after 28 days of life). However, continuous fetal heart rate monitoring is associated with a significant increase in obstetric intervention, including operative vaginal and cesarean delivery.

7. According to the 2008 NICHD Workshop Report on EFM, a "Category II" fetal heart rate tracing is one that falls between "Category I" and "Category III." It is an EFM tracing that is not formally reactive, but is reassuring. It is also referred to as suspicious, equivocal or indeterminate. It is the most common type of tracing, and can be seen in up to 60% of labors, suggesting that it is not specific to fetal hypoxia. A "Category II" tracing at term is associated with poor perinatal outcome in only 20% of cases. The significance of such a tracing depends on the clinical endpoint. If the end-point is a 5 min Apgar score <7, then it has a sensitivity of 50–60% and positive predictive value of 10–15% (assuming a prevalence of 4%). If the end-point of interest is permanent cerebral injury, then it has a 99.9% false-positive rate.

8. Interventions to improve EFW performance include discontinuation of oxytocin infusion, repositioning the patient (in an effort to improve venous return), oxygen supplementation by facemask, and intravenous fluid infusion.

9. Fetal scalp sampling refers to sampling of capillary blood from the fetal scalp during labor to measure pH. Capillary pH lies between that of arterial and venous blood. This technique was introduced by Saling in 1962, and is most useful in labor when alternative noninvasive tests are unable to confirm fetal well-being. Suggested management based on fetal scalp pH is as follows: (i) pH >7.25, continue expectant management; (ii) pH 7.20–7.25, repeat at 20–30 min intervals until delivery; and (iii) ph <7.20, proceed with immediate and urgent delivery.

10. According to the 2008 NICHD Workshop Report on EFM, a "Category III" fetal heart rate tracing is one that is ominous and requires immediate action. It is also referred to as nonreassuring. It occurs in only 0.3% of intrapartum fetal heart rate tracings, but is associated with adverse events in over 50% of cases. It is characterized by absent fetal heart rate variability (defined as peak-to-trough excursions of 0 bpm around the baseline), absence of accelerations, and repetitive late or severe variable decelerations. Decelerations are regarded as "repetitive" if they occur with more than 50% of contractions.

60 Cesarean Delivery[1]

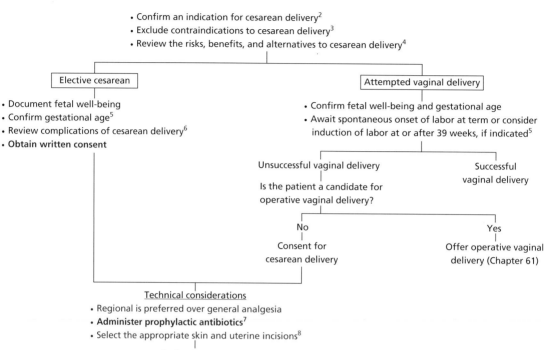

- Confirm an indication for cesarean delivery[2]
- Exclude contraindications to cesarean delivery[3]
- Review the risks, benefits, and alternatives to cesarean delivery[4]

Elective cesarean

- Document fetal well-being
- Confirm gestational age[5]
- Review complications of cesarean delivery[6]
- **Obtain written consent**

Attempted vaginal delivery

- Confirm fetal well-being and gestational age
- Await spontaneous onset of labor at term or consider induction of labor at or after 39 weeks, if indicated[5]

Unsuccessful vaginal delivery

Is the patient a candidate for operative vaginal delivery?

Successful vaginal delivery

No
Consent for cesarean delivery

Yes
Offer operative vaginal delivery (Chapter 61)

Technical considerations
- Regional is preferred over general analgesia
- **Administer prophylactic antibiotics[7]**
- Select the appropriate skin and uterine incisions[8]

Postpartum care
- Early ambulation
- Prophylactic anticoagulation, if indicated
- Observe for complications[6]
- **Pain management**

Review the options for delivery in a subsequent pregnancy[9]

1. Cesarean delivery refers to delivery of a fetus via the abdominal route (laparotomy) requiring an incision into the uterus (hysterotomy). It is the second most common surgical procedure (behind male circumcision), accounting for 25–30% of all deliveries in the US.

2. Most indications for cesarean are relative and rely on the judgment of the obstetric care provider. *Absolute indications* for cesarean include a prior high vertical ("classic")

cesarean, complete placenta previa, absolute cephalopelvic disproportion (CPD) (where the disparity between the size of the bony pelvis and the fetal head precludes vaginal delivery even under optimal conditions), prior full-thickness myomectomy, prior uterine rupture, malpresentation (transverse lie), cord prolapse (Chapter 73), active genital HSV infection in labor, and nonreassuring fetal testing ("fetal distress") prior to labor. *Relative indications* include a prior low transverse hysterotomy, labor

Obstetric Clinical Algorithms: Management and Evidence. By © E.R. Norwitz, M. Belfort, G.R. Saade and H. Miller.
Published 2010 Blackwell Publishing.

dystocia (failure to progress in labor), breech presentation, relative CPD, multiple pregnancy, women with certain cardiac or cerebrovascular disease, select fetal anomalies (such as hydrocephalus), maternal request, and excessive hemorrhage at delivery (puerperal hysterectomy is a highly morbid procedure and should only be performed as a last resort to save the life of the mother). A desire for permanent sterilization (tubal ligation) is not an adequate indication for cesarean delivery.

3. Contraindications to cesarean delivery include uncontrolled maternal coagulopathy and failure to obtain maternal consent.

4. The most common indication for a primary cesarean is failure to progress in labor, which is defined as abnormal or inadequate progress in labor. Causes include the 3 Ps: inadequate "powers" (uterine contractions), inadequate "passage" (bony pelvis) or abnormalities of the "passenger" (fetal macrosomia, hydrocephalus, malpresentation). If contractions are "adequate," one of two events will occur: dilation and effacement of the cervix with descent of the head or worsening caput succedaneum (scalp edema) and molding (overlapping of the skull bones). If contractions are inadequate, consider augmentation with pitocin infusion with or without an intrauterine pressure catheter (IUPC).

5. Elective cesarean delivery should only be performed at or after 39 weeks, with the exception of HIV and twins where it can be performed at or after 38 weeks. Elective delivery prior to these gestational ages should only be performed after documentation of fetal lung maturity.

6. Complications of cesarean include excessive bleeding, infection, venous thromboembolic disease, injury to adjacent organs (bladder, bowel, ureters), and (rarely) injury to the fetus.

7. Routine use of broad-spectrum prophylactic antibiotics given 20–30 minutes prior to surgery (and not after clamping of the cord after delivery) will decrease the incidence of postoperative febrile morbidity. Penicillin for GBS chemoprophylaxis is not sufficient to prevent wound infection.

8. Skin incision may be either Pfannenstiel (low transverse incision, muscle separating, strong but limited exposure) or midline vertical (offers the best exposure but is weak). Pfannenstiel incisions may be modified to improve exposure, if needed, by dividing the rectus muscles horizontally (Maylard incision) or lifting the rectus off the pubic bone (Cherney incision). Pfannenstiel should be the incision of choice. Similarly, a low transverse hysterotomy should be performed, if possible. Indications for high vertical ("classic") hysterotomy include extreme prematurity, breech presentation, multiple pregnancy, and failure to gain access to the lower uterine segment due, for example, to excessive adhesions. Elective surgery (such as myomectomy) should not be performed at the time of caesarean, because of the risk of bleeding.

9. A prior high vertical ("classic") cesarean, a prior low vertical cesarean, and two or more low transverse hysterotomies should be regarded as an absolute contraindication to attempted vaginal delivery, because of the risk of uterine dehiscence and rupture. Uterine rupture may be life-threatening. Symptoms and signs include acute onset of fetal bradycardia (70%), abdominal pain (10%), vaginal bleeding (5%), hemodynamic instability (5–10%), and/or loss of the presenting part (<5%). In such women, repeat cesarean should be performed at or after 36 weeks after confirmation of fetal lung maturity. Vaginal birth after caesarean (VBAC) (see Chapter 54) may be a reasonable alternative for elective repeat cesarean delivery in selected patients so long as certain criteria are fulfilled, including: no induction of labor (especially with prostaglandins), continuous fetal heart rate monitoring, adequate analgesia, careful monitoring of the progress of labor to facilitate the early diagnosis of CPD, and immediate access to emergency cesarean. A successful VBAC can be achieved in 65–80% of women.

61 Operative Vaginal Delivery[1]

- **Confirm an indication for operative vaginal delivery[2]**
- **Exclude contraindications to operative vaginal delivery[3]**
- **Be aware of the type of operative vaginal delivery you will be performing[4]**
- Review the risks, benefits, and alternatives to operative vaginal delivery
- Discuss potential complications to the mother and fetus[5]

Ensure that all prerequisites for operative vaginal delivery have been fulfilled			
Maternal criteria	Fetal criteria	Uteroplacental criteria	Other criteria
• Adequate analgesia • Lithotomy position • Bladder empty • Clinical pelvimetry must be adequate in dimension and size to facilitate an atraumatic delivery • Verbal or written consent	• Vertex presentation • Fetal head must be engaged in pelvis • Position of fetal head must be known • Station of fetal head must be ≥ +2 • Attitude of fetal head and presence of caput succedaneum and/or molding should be noted	• Cervix fully dilated • Membranes ruptured • No placenta previa	• Experienced operator who is fully acquainted with the use of the instrument • The capability to perform an emergency cesarean delivery if required

≥45° rotation required
Use rotational forceps (Kiellands, Barton forceps)

Vertex presentation, no rotation or rotation <45° required
Use "classic" forceps (Simpson, Tucker-McLane, Elliot forceps) OR vacuum extractor (Ventouse)[6]

Aftercoming head in a vaginal breech delivery
Use forceps designed to assist in breech deliveries (Piper forceps)

Technical considerations
- **Ensure correct placement of the forceps[7] or vacuum[8]**
- Apply traction in concert with maternal expulsive efforts

Successful operative vaginal delivery
Examine the fetus and maternal perineum for evidence of injury

Unsuccessful operative vaginal delivery[9]
Proceed with cesarean delivery (no place for combined forceps and vaginal delivery)

1. Operative vaginal delivery refers to any operative procedure designed to expedite vaginal delivery, including forceps delivery and vacuum extraction.

2. Indications for operative vaginal delivery include: (i) *maternal indications* such as maternal exhaustion, inadequate maternal expulsive efforts (women with spinal cord injuries or neuromuscular diseases), need to avoid maternal expulsive efforts (women with certain cardiac or cerebrovascular disease); (ii) *fetal indications* such as nonreassuring

fetal testing ("fetal distress"); and (iii) *other indications* such as prolonged second stage of labor (nullipara: ≥2 hours without regional analgesia, ≥3 hours with regional analgesia; multipara: ≥1 hour without regional analgesia, ≥2 hours with regional analgesia), elective shortening of the second stage of labor using outlet forceps.

3. Contraindications to operative vaginal delivery include placenta previa, absolute cephalopelvic disproportion or any other contraindication to vaginal delivery; prematurity

Obstetric Clinical Algorithms: Management and Evidence. By © E.R. Norwitz, M. Belfort, G.R. Saade and H. Miller.
Published 2010 Blackwell Publishing.

(gestational age <34 weeks is an absolute contraindication for vacuum but not forceps delivery); suspected fetal skeletal dysplasia; suspected fetal coagulation disorder; fetal macrosomia (a relative contraindication); or failure to fulfill the prerequisites listed in the table (such as station >2+ , intact membranes, cervix not fully dilated or failure to obtain consent).

4. The 1988 ACOG classification of forceps deliveries is outlined in Table 61.1 . The old category of "high forceps" (in which forceps were placed with the fetal head floating and ballottable above the brim of the true pelvis) has been abandoned due to excessive fetal risk. Mid-forceps deliveries should be performed only by competent operators, and after careful consideration of alternative approaches (oxytocin administration, cesarean or continued expectant management) and of the potential fetal risks. Indications for vacuum extraction-assisted delivery are similar to those for forceps delivery.

5. Potential complications of operative vaginal delivery include maternal perineal injury (especially with rotational forceps delivery) and fetal complications such as facial bruising, laceration, and cephalhematoma (more common with vacuum extraction). Facial nerve palsy, skull fractures, cervical spine injuries, and intracranial hemorrhage are rare. Failed operative vaginal delivery is more common with vacuum than with forceps, and more common with the soft cup vacuum extractor that with the rigid "M" cup.

6. There is no proven benefit of one instrument over another. The choice of which instrument to use depends largely on clinician preference and experience. In some circumstances, one instrument may be preferred over another. For example, vacuum extraction can be accomplished with minimal maternal analgesia.

7. Exact knowledge of fetal position, station, and degree of asynclitism (lateral flexion) is essential to proper forceps application. After performing a "phantom application," the right forceps blade (left handle) is placed followed by the left forceps blade. The handles are then locked. Proper application is determined by assessing the position of the forceps relative to three landmarks on the fetal skull: the posterior fontanelle, sagittal suture, and parietal bones. If rotation is required, it should be performed at this time. Delivery is then accomplished by traction applied along the pelvic curve in concert with uterine contractions.

8. To promote flexion of the fetal head with descent, the suction cup of the vacuum should be placed over the "median flexing point" (i.e. symmetrically astride the sagittal suture with the posterior margin of the cup 1–3 cm anterior to the posterior fontanelle). Low suction (100 mmHg) should be applied. After ensuring that no maternal soft tissue is trapped between the cup and fetal head, suction should be increased to 500–600 mmHg and sustained downward traction applied along the pelvic curve in concert with uterine contractions. Suction is released between contractions. Ideally, episiotomy should be avoided as pressure of the perineum on the vacuum cup will help to keep it applied to the fetal head and assist in flexion and rotation.

9. The procedure should be abandoned if the vacuum cup detaches three times, if there is no descent of the fetal head or if delivery is not effected within 30 minutes.

Table 61.1 ACOG classification of forceps deliveries

Type of procedure	Criteria
Outlet forceps	1. Scalp is visible at the introitus without separating the labia 2. Fetal skull has reached the level of the pelvic floor 3. Sagittal suture is in the direct anteroposterior diameter or in the right or left occiput anterior or posterior position 4. Fetal head is at or on the perineum 5. Rotation is ≤45°
Low forceps	Leading point of the fetal skull (station) is station +2 or more but has not yet reached the pelvic floor
Mid-forceps	The head is engaged in the pelvis but the presenting part is above +2 station
High forceps	(Not included in this classification)

62 Intrapartum Management of Twin Pregnancy

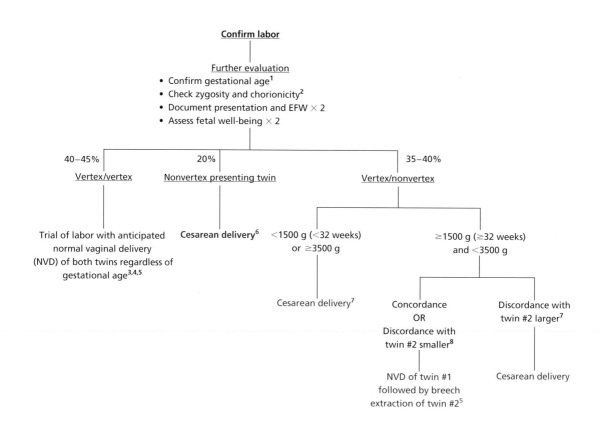

Confirm labor

Further evaluation
- Confirm gestational age[1]
- Check zygosity and chorionicity[2]
- Document presentation and EFW × 2
- Assess fetal well-being × 2

40–45%
Vertex/vertex

Trial of labor with anticipated normal vaginal delivery (NVD) of both twins regardless of gestational age[3,4,5]

20%
Nonvertex presenting twin

Cesarean delivery[6]

35–40%
Vertex/nonvertex

<1500 g (<32 weeks) or ≥3500 g

Cesarean delivery[7]

≥1500 g (≥32 weeks) and <3500 g

Concordance
OR
Discordance with twin #2 smaller[8]

NVD of twin #1 followed by breech extraction of twin #2[5]

Discordance with twin #2 larger[7]

Cesarean delivery

Obstetric Clinical Algorithms: Management and Evidence. By © E.R. Norwitz, M. Belfort, G.R. Saade and H. Miller.
Published 2010 Blackwell Publishing.

1. There is considerable controversy about the intrapartum management of twin pregnancies, which is due primarily to an absence of well-designed clinical trials and to conflicting recommendations in the literature. It is generally recommended that diamniotic twin pregnancies be delivered by 40 weeks. If an <u>elective</u> delivery of twins is planned prior to 38 weeks, ACOG requires that fetal lung maturity be documented. It is generally acceptable to obtain amniotic fluid from only one sac (traditionally the nonpresenting twin) for assessment of fetal pulmonary maturity. However, if there is discordant growth between the fetuses, it is recommended that both sacs be sampled.

2. Monoamniotic twin pregnancies should be delivered by elective cesarean at 32–34 weeks, because of the risk of fetal demise secondary to cord entanglement.

3. Continuous electronic fetal monitoring of both fetuses is required throughout labor and delivery. Intravenous access should be attained and blood readily available, if needed. Anesthesiology should be notified and regional anesthesia recommended. Cesarean delivery may be indicated for the usual obstetric indications (such as non-reassuring fetal testing, placenta previa or elective repeat cesarean after prior cesarean delivery). It is generally recommended that a neonatologist be present at delivery, because a second twin is more likely to require resuscitation. If a vaginal delivery is to be attempted, ultrasound equipment should be available throughout labor and delivery to document the fetal heart rate of the second twin, if necessary, and to confirm presentation (note that presentation of the second twin may change in up to 20% of cases after delivery of twin #1). With the possible exception of concordant, vertex/vertex, diamniotic twin pregnancies in labor at term, all twin pregnancies should be delivered in the operating room with the availability of urgent cesarean delivery.

4. Internal podalic version and breech extraction of twin #2 is an acceptable option. An obstetrician skilled in operative vaginal delivery and vaginal breech delivery is a prerequisite for any such delivery.

5. In the setting of reassuring intrapartum fetal heart rate monitoring, there is no urgency to deliver twin #2, since delivery interval *per se* does <u>not</u> appear to affect perinatal outcome. However, a delivery interval of >15 min is associated with an increased risk of cesarean delivery. For this reason, active rather than expectant management of the second twin (artificial rupture of membranes, oxytocin augmentation, and/or breech extraction) is generally recommended.

6. There is no place for external cephalic version of twin #1.

7. Cesarean delivery is commonly recommended in this setting to avoid breech vaginal delivery of twin #2 (although several studies have suggested that vaginal breech delivery of fetuses <1500 g may be safe).

8. Discordance is defined as ≥25% difference between twins. It is calculated using the following formula: EFW of larger fetus – EFW of smaller fetus/EFW of larger fetus, and is usually expressed as a %.

63 Postpartum Hemorrhage[1]

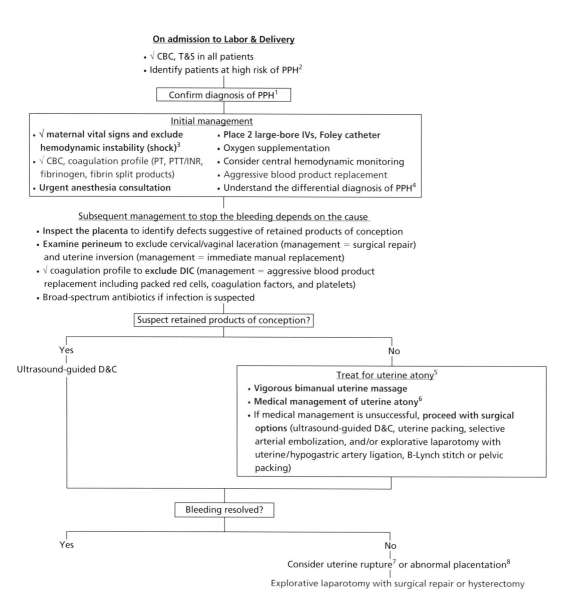

On admission to Labor & Delivery
- √ CBC, T&S in all patients
- Identify patients at high risk of PPH[2]

Confirm diagnosis of PPH[1]

Initial management
- √ maternal vital signs and exclude hemodynamic instability (shock)[3]
- √ CBC, coagulation profile (PT, PTT/INR, fibrinogen, fibrin split products)
- Urgent anesthesia consultation
- Place 2 large-bore IVs, Foley catheter
- Oxygen supplementation
- Consider central hemodynamic monitoring
- Aggressive blood product replacement
- Understand the differential diagnosis of PPH[4]

Subsequent management to stop the bleeding depends on the cause
- **Inspect the placenta** to identify defects suggestive of retained products of conception
- **Examine perineum** to exclude cervical/vaginal laceration (management = surgical repair) and uterine inversion (management = immediate manual replacement)
- √ coagulation profile to **exclude DIC** (management = aggressive blood product replacement including packed red cells, coagulation factors, and platelets)
- Broad-spectrum antibiotics if infection is suspected

Suspect retained products of conception?

Yes
Ultrasound-guided D&C

No

Treat for uterine atony[5]
- Vigorous bimanual uterine massage
- Medical management of uterine atony[6]
- If medical management is unsuccessful, **proceed with surgical options** (ultrasound-guided D&C, uterine packing, selective arterial embolization, and/or explorative laparotomy with uterine/hypogastric artery ligation, B-Lynch stitch or pelvic packing)

Bleeding resolved?

Yes

No
Consider uterine rupture[7] or abnormal placentation[8]
Explorative laparotomy with surgical repair or hysterectomy

Obstetric Clinical Algorithms: Management and Evidence. By © E.R. Norwitz, M. Belfort, G.R. Saade and H. Miller. Published 2010 Blackwell Publishing.

1. Hemorrhage is the third most common cause of maternal mortality (after thromboembolic disease and pre-eclampsia). *Postpartum hemorrhage (PPH)* has traditionally been defined as an estimated blood loss (EBL) of ≥500 mL at vaginal delivery. However, clinicians typically underestimate blood loss by 30–50%. The average blood loss following vaginal delivery is 500 mL, with 5% of women losing >1000 mL. Blood loss at cesarean averages 1000 mL. More recently, PPH has been defined as a 10% drop in hematocrit from admission or bleeding requiring blood transfusion. Using this definition, PPH complicates 4% of vaginal deliveries and 6–8% of cesarean deliveries.

2. Risk factors for PPH include a prior history of PPH, grand multiparity, fetal macrosomia, multiple pregnancy, known coagulopathy, pre-eclampsia, obesity, intra-amniotic infection, uterine relaxant drugs (magnesium sulfate, nitrates), prolonged second stage of labor, precipitate delivery, and cesarean and operative vaginal delivery. In patients at high risk of PPH, consider type and cross blood products and early anesthesia consultation. If massive PPH is suspected prior to delivery (for example, placenta increta/percreta), consider planning elective cesarean with general surgery back-up with or without preoperative uterine artery balloon catheter placement.

3. In general, pregnant women are young, with an increased circulating blood volume. They are therefore somewhat protected against excessive blood loss. Blood loss of <900 mL (<15% of blood volume) produces few symptoms. Blood loss of 1200–1500 mL (20–25%) will cause orthostasis; blood loss of 1200–1500 mL (30–35%) will be evident as hypotension; and blood loss >2400 mL (>40%) is required before hypovolemic shock will develop.

4. Postpartum hemorrhage is classified as early (defined as PPH <24 hours after delivery) or late (>24 hours but <6 weeks postpartum). Causes of early PPH include uterine atony, retained placental fragments, lower genital tract lacerations, uterine rupture, uterine inversion, and abnormal placentation. Late PPH is more likely to be due to retained placental fragments, infection (endometritis), and coagulopathy.

5. *Uterine atony* is the most common cause of PPH. Risk factors include uterine overdistension (due to polyhydramnios, multiple pregnancy, fetal macrosomia), high parity, rapid or prolonged labor, infection, prior uterine atony, and use of uterine-relaxing agents.

6. Medical management of uterine atony includes the following.
- *Oxytocin* 10–40 units in 1 L normal saline or Ringer's lactate given by continuous iv infusion. Can be given im. Side-effects may include nausea and vomiting and water intoxication.
- *Methylergonovine (methergine)* 0.2 mg im or imm (never iv) every 2–4 hours. Side-effects may include nausea and vomiting and vasospasm (hypertension and myocardial ischemia). Contraindications include hypertension and coronary insufficiency.
- *Hemabate (carboprost)* $(PGF_2\alpha)$ 0.25 mg im or imm every 15–90 minutes for a maximum of eight doses. Side-effects may include nausea and vomiting, diarrhea, flushing, fever, vasospasm, and bronchospasm. Contraindications include cardiac, pulmonary, renal, and hepatic disease.
- *Dinoprostone (PGE2)* 20 mg vaginally, orally or rectally every 2 hours. Side-effects may include nausea and vomiting, diarrhea, headache, fever, and vasodilation. Hypotension is a contraindication.
- *Misoprostil (PGE1)* 1000 μg rectally. Side-effects are rare.

7. *Uterine rupture* is a rare but dangerous cause of PPH, complicating 1 in 2000 deliveries. Risk factors include prior uterine surgery (cesarean), obstructed labor, "excessive" use of oxytocin, abnormal fetal lie, grand multiparity, and uterine manipulations in labor (forceps delivery, breech extraction, and intrauterine pressure catheter insertion). Treatment is explorative laparotomy with surgical repair or hysterectomy.

8. *Abnormal placentation* includes abnormal attachment of placental villi to the myometrium (accreta), invasion into the myometrium (increta) or penetration through the myometrium (percreta). Risk factors include prior uterine surgery (cesarean), placenta previa, smoking, and grand multiparity. Placenta previa alone is associated with a 5% incidence of accreta, which increases to 10–25% with placenta previa and one prior cesarean, and >50% with placenta previa and two or more prior cesareans. Management is D&C or explorative laparotomy with surgical repair or hysterectomy.

64 Retained Placenta

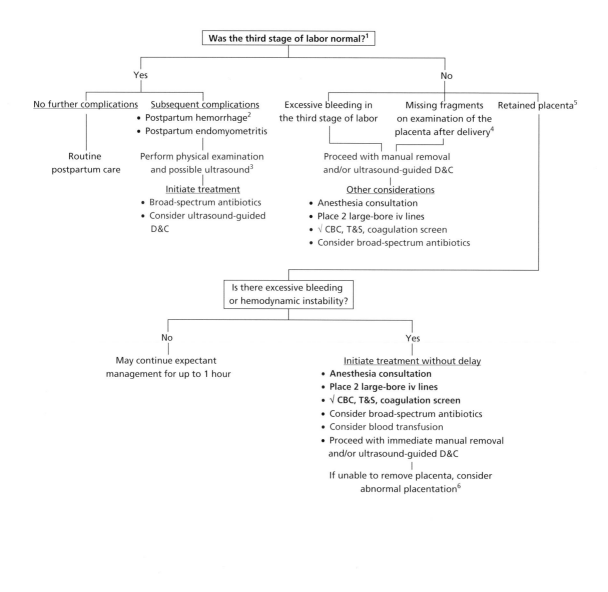

Was the third stage of labor normal?[1]

Yes

No further complications

Routine postpartum care

Subsequent complications
- Postpartum hemorrhage[2]
- Postpartum endomyometritis

Perform physical examination and possible ultrasound[3]

Initiate treatment
- Broad-spectrum antibiotics
- Consider ultrasound-guided D&C

No

Excessive bleeding in the third stage of labor

Missing fragments on examination of the placenta after delivery[4]

Retained placenta[5]

Proceed with manual removal and/or ultrasound-guided D&C

Other considerations
- Anesthesia consultation
- Place 2 large-bore iv lines
- √ CBC, T&S, coagulation screen
- Consider broad-spectrum antibiotics

Is there excessive bleeding or hemodynamic instability?

No

May continue expectant management for up to 1 hour

Yes

Initiate treatment without delay
- **Anesthesia consultation**
- **Place 2 large-bore iv lines**
- **√ CBC, T&S, coagulation screen**
- Consider broad-spectrum antibiotics
- Consider blood transfusion
- Proceed with immediate manual removal and/or ultrasound-guided D&C

If unable to remove placenta, consider abnormal placentation[6]

Obstetric Clinical Algorithms: Management and Evidence. By © E.R. Norwitz, M. Belfort, G.R. Saade and H. Miller.
Published 2010 Blackwell Publishing.

1. The third stage of labor begins with delivery of the fetus and ends with delivery of the placenta and fetal membranes. It is usually managed expectantly. Uterine contractions result in cleavage of the placenta between the zona basalis and zona spongiosum. The three clinical signs of placental separation are: (i) a gush of blood ("separation bleed"); (ii) apparent lengthening of the umbilical cord; and (iii) elevation and contraction of the uterine fundus. Placental separation can be encouraged – also known as active management of the third stage of labor – by "controlled cord traction" using either the Brandt–Andrews maneuver (where the uterus is secured and controlled traction is applied to the cord) or the Credé maneuver (where the cord is secured and the uterus is elevated). The mean duration of the third stage of labor is 6 minutes.

2. Postpartum hemorrhage (PPH) has traditionally been defined as an estimated blood loss of ≥500 mL. However, blood loss is underestimated clinically by 30–50%. The average blood loss following vaginal delivery is 500 mL, with 5% of women losing >1000 mL. Blood loss following cesarean averages 1000 mL. More recently, PPH has been defined as a 10% drop in hematocrit from admission or bleeding requiring blood transfusion (see Chapter 63). Retained placental fragments is one cause of PPH.

3. A careful physical examination (including a bimanual examination) should be performed in all such women. Evidence of vaginal bleeding with an open cervical os suggests retained placental fragments and/or blood clots. Although an ultrasound examination is often performed in such women, management should be based primarily on their clinical presentation. Indeed, the definition of what constitutes a normal postpartum ultrasound is not clear.

4. The placenta and fetal membranes should be carefully examined after every delivery. Such an examination may identify defects suggestive of retained placental fragments, including retention of a cotyledon or succenturiate lobe that is seen in 3% of placentae.

5. Retained placenta is defined as failure of the placenta and fetal membranes to deliver within 30 minutes of delivery of the baby, which complicates 3–5% of all deliveries. If there is excessive bleeding, manual removal and/or D&C may be required earlier.

6. See Chapter 45.

65 Postpartum Endomyometritis[1]

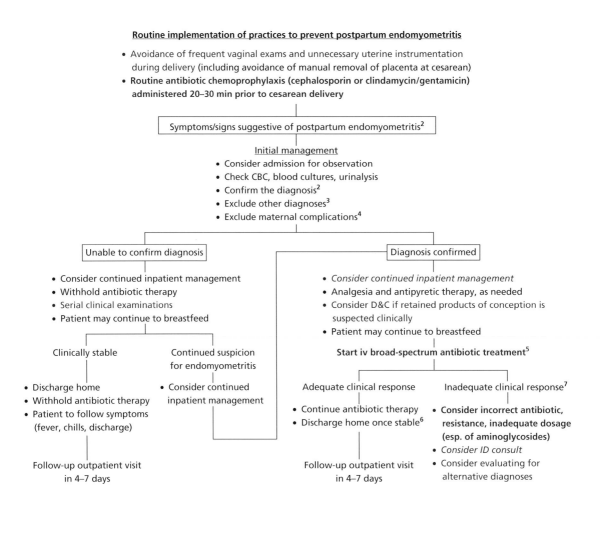

Routine implementation of practices to prevent postpartum endomyometritis

- Avoidance of frequent vaginal exams and unnecessary uterine instrumentation during delivery (including avoidance of manual removal of placenta at cesarean)
- **Routine antibiotic chemoprophylaxis (cephalosporin or clindamycin/gentamicin) administered 20–30 min prior to cesarean delivery**

Symptoms/signs suggestive of postpartum endomyometritis[2]

Initial management
- Consider admission for observation
- Check CBC, blood cultures, urinalysis
- Confirm the diagnosis[2]
- Exclude other diagnoses[3]
- Exclude maternal complications[4]

Unable to confirm diagnosis

- Consider continued inpatient management
- Withhold antibiotic therapy
- Serial clinical examinations
- Patient may continue to breastfeed

Clinically stable

- Discharge home
- Withhold antibiotic therapy
- Patient to follow symptoms (fever, chills, discharge)

Follow-up outpatient visit in 4–7 days

Continued suspicion for endomyometritis

- Consider continued inpatient management

Diagnosis confirmed

- *Consider continued inpatient management*
- Analgesia and antipyretic therapy, as needed
- Consider D&C if retained products of conception is suspected clinically
- Patient may continue to breastfeed

Start iv broad-spectrum antibiotic treatment[5]

Adequate clinical response

- Continue antibiotic therapy
- Discharge home once stable[6]

Follow-up outpatient visit in 4–7 days

Inadequate clinical response[7]

- **Consider incorrect antibiotic, resistance, inadequate dosage (esp. of aminoglycosides)**
- *Consider ID consult*
- Consider evaluating for alternative diagnoses

Obstetric Clinical Algorithms: Management and Evidence. By © E.R. Norwitz, M. Belfort, G.R. Saade and H. Miller.
Published 2010 Blackwell Publishing.

1. Postpartum endomyometritis refers to a polymicrobial infection of uterine cavity following delivery. It complicates approximately 6–8% of all deliveries. Risk factors for postpartum endomyometritis include cesarean delivery, prolonged rupture of the fetal membranes (>24 h), low socio-economic status, diabetes, multiple vaginal examinations, manual removal of the placenta, and internal fetal monitoring.

2. Postpartum endomyometritis is a <u>clinical</u> diagnosis characterized by fever, uterine tenderness, a foul purulent vaginal discharge, and/or an increase in vaginal bleeding during the puerperium. It occurs most commonly 5–10 days after delivery. Constitutional symptoms (chills, malaise) and an elevated white cell count are common findings, but are not required for the diagnosis. There is no place for radiologic imaging studies or culture of the endometrial cavity to confirm the diagnosis; however, imaging studies may be useful to exclude other possible diagnoses (such as retained placental tissue or septic pelvic thrombophlebitis).

3. The differential diagnosis of postpartum endomyometritis includes retained products of conception, mastitis, septic pelvic thrombophlebitis, pelvic/bladder flap hematoma or abscess, wound or episiotomy infection, and other infections (such as appendicitis, pyelonephritis, and pneumonia).

4. Maternal complications include necrotizing fasciitis, pulmonary edema, sepsis, adult respiratory distress syndrome (ARDS), and subsequent Asherman syndrome (especially following uterine instrumentation).

5. Prompt administration of intravenous broad-spectrum antibiotics will reduce maternal febrile morbidity and duration of hospitalization. Intravenous ampicillin 2 g q 6 h plus gentamicin 1.5 mg/kg q 8 h (after confirmation of normal renal function) are the antibiotics of choice following vaginal delivery. After cesarean delivery, clindamycin 900 mg iv q 8 h should be added. If an abscess is suspected or renal impairment develops, aztreonam can be substituted for gentamicin.

6. Intravenous antibiotics should be continued until the patient is 24–48 hours afebrile and asymptomatic. There is no role for oral antibiotics once the patient is discharged (aside from patients with positive blood cultures who likely require antibiotics for a total of 10–14 days).

7. Ten percent of patients with symptomatic postpartum endomyometritis will fail to respond to intravenous antibiotics within 48–72 hours; 20% will be due to resistant organisms. Consider evaluating for other sources of infection such as pyelonephritis, abscess or septic pelvic thrombophlebitis.

66 Mastitis[1]

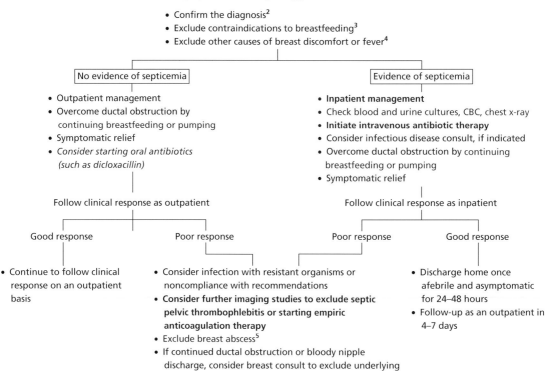

Symptoms and/or signs suggestive of mastitis

- Confirm the diagnosis[2]
- Exclude contraindications to breastfeeding[3]
- Exclude other causes of breast discomfort or fever[4]

No evidence of septicemia

- Outpatient management
- Overcome ductal obstruction by continuing breastfeeding or pumping
- Symptomatic relief
- *Consider starting oral antibiotics (such as dicloxacillin)*

Follow clinical response as outpatient

Good response

- Continue to follow clinical response on an outpatient basis

Poor response

- Consider infection with resistant organisms or noncompliance with recommendations
- **Consider further imaging studies to exclude septic pelvic thrombophlebitis or starting empiric anticoagulation therapy**
- Exclude breast abscess[5]
- If continued ductal obstruction or bloody nipple discharge, consider breast consult to exclude underlying mass lesion/malignancy

Evidence of septicemia

- **Inpatient management**
- Check blood and urine cultures, CBC, chest x-ray
- **Initiate intravenous antibiotic therapy**
- Consider infectious disease consult, if indicated
- Overcome ductal obstruction by continuing breastfeeding or pumping
- Symptomatic relief

Follow clinical response as inpatient

Poor response

Good response

- Discharge home once afebrile and asymptomatic for 24–48 hours
- Follow-up as an outpatient in 4–7 days

Obstetric Clinical Algorithms: Management and Evidence. By © E.R. Norwitz, M. Belfort, G.R. Saade and H. Miller.
Published 2010 Blackwell Publishing.

1. Mastitis refers to a regional infection of the breast parenchyma, usually by *Staphylococcus aureus*.

2. Mastitis is a clinical diagnosis with fever, chills, and focal unilateral breast erythema, edema, and tenderness with or without an elevated white blood cell count. It is more common in primiparous patients (>50%) and usually occurs during the third or fourth week postpartum.

3. Whenever possible, breastfeeding should be encouraged. Breastfed infants have a lower incidence of allergies, gastrointestinal infections, ear infections, respiratory infections, and (possibly) higher intelligence quotient (IQ) scores. Women who breastfeed appear to have a lower incidence of breast cancer, ovarian cancer, and osteoporosis. Breastfeeding is also a bonding experience between infant and mother. Under certain conditions, however, breastfeeding may be detrimental to the fetus. Contraindications to breastfeeding include infection with HIV, cytomegalovirus, and/or (more controversially) chronic hepatitis B and C. Breastfeeding is also contraindicated if the mother is on certain drugs, such as radioisotopes and certain cytotoxic agents.

4. Mastitis should be distinguished from breast engorgement, which typically occurs on days 2–4 postpartum in women who are not nursing or at any time if breastfeeding is interrupted. Conservative measures (tight top, ice packs, analgesics) are usually effective for the management of breast engorgement, although bromocriptine may be indicated in refractory cases. Other causes of fever that should be excluded in the puerperium include endometritis, urinary tract infection/pyelonephritis, ear and throat infections, pneumonia, and (rarely) septic pelvic thrombophlebitis.

5. Approximately 5–10% of women will develop a breast abscess. Diagnosis can be made clinically and confirmed by ultrasonography, if indicated. Treatment is adequate surgical drainage.

67 Vasa Previa

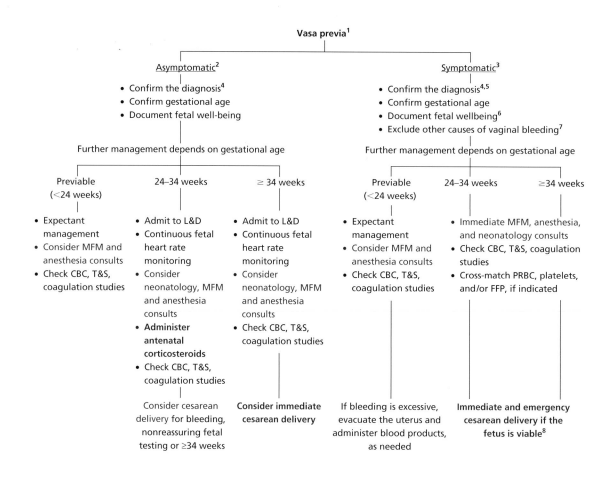

Vasa previa[1]

Asymptomatic[2]
- Confirm the diagnosis[4]
- Confirm gestational age
- Document fetal well-being

Further management depends on gestational age

Previable (<24 weeks)
- Expectant management
- Consider MFM and anesthesia consults
- Check CBC, T&S, coagulation studies

24–34 weeks
- Admit to L&D
- Continuous fetal heart rate monitoring
- Consider neonatology, MFM and anesthesia consults
- **Administer antenatal corticosteroids**
- Check CBC, T&S, coagulation studies

Consider cesarean delivery for bleeding, nonreassuring fetal testing or ≥34 weeks

≥ 34 weeks
- Admit to L&D
- Continuous fetal heart rate monitoring
- Consider neonatology, MFM and anesthesia consults
- Check CBC, T&S, coagulation studies

Consider immediate cesarean delivery

Symptomatic[3]
- Confirm the diagnosis[4,5]
- Confirm gestational age
- Document fetal wellbeing[6]
- Exclude other causes of vaginal bleeding[7]

Further management depends on gestational age

Previable (<24 weeks)
- Expectant management
- Consider MFM and anesthesia consults
- Check CBC, T&S, coagulation studies

If bleeding is excessive, evacuate the uterus and administer blood products, as needed

24–34 weeks
- Immediate MFM, anesthesia, and neonatology consults
- Check CBC, T&S, coagulation studies
- Cross-match PRBC, platelets, and/or FFP, if indicated

≥34 weeks

Immediate and emergency cesarean delivery if the fetus is viable[8]

Obstetric Clinical Algorithms: Management and Evidence. By © E.R. Norwitz, M. Belfort, G.R. Saade and H. Miller.
Published 2010 Blackwell Publishing.

1. Vasa previa refers to fetal vessels coursing through the membranes (velamentous insertion) overlying the internal os ahead of the presenting part of the fetus.

2. Vasa previa may be an incidental finding on routine ultrasound.

3. Symptoms typically include the acute onset of bright-red vaginal bleeding, which is usually painless. It is often accompanied by decreased fetal movement. Risks for bleeding from fetal blood vessels include rupture of the fetal membranes, funic (cord) presentation, multiple pregnancy, placental abnormalities (such as an accessory or succenturiate lobe of placenta, velamentous cord insertion).

4. Vasa previa is an ultrasonographic diagnosis. Ultrasound may confirm funic presentation with or without velamentous cord insertion.

5. In the setting of acute bleeding, perform a bedside Apt test (hemoglobin alkaline denaturation test). This involves addition of 2–3 drops of an alkaline solution (sodium or potassium hydroxide) to 1 mL of blood collected from a vaginal pool. If blood is maternal, erythrocytes rupture and the mixture turns brown. However, fetal erythrocytes are resistant to rupture and the mixture remains red. Certain maternal conditions (hemoglobinopathies) may give false-positive test.

6. Maternal complications are rare. The bleeding is fetal in origin. As such, fetal mortality is $\geq 75\%$ due primarily to fetal exsanguination. Perinatal outcome depends primarily on the extent of the fetal bleeding, the gestational age, and the ability of the obstetric care provider to make the diagnosis and expedite delivery.

7. Other causes of vaginal bleeding include placenta previa, placental abruption, early labor, and genital tract lesions (cervical polyps or erosions).

8. Contraindications to emergency cesarean include a previable fetus (<24 weeks), intrauterine fetal demise, maternal hemodynamic instability or coagulopathy, or failure to obtain maternal consent for surgery.

68 Postpartum Psychiatric Disorders

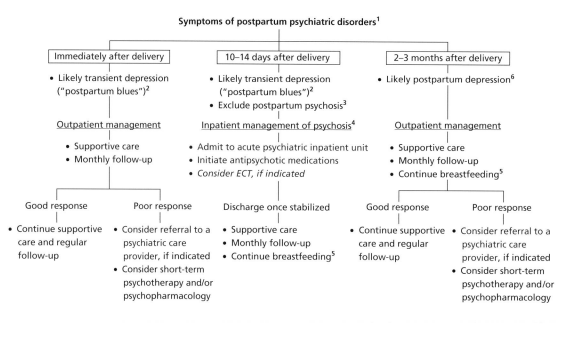

Symptoms of postpartum psychiatric disorders[1]

Immediately after delivery

- Likely transient depression ("postpartum blues")[2]

Outpatient management

- Supportive care
- Monthly follow-up

Good response

- Continue supportive care and regular follow-up

Poor response

- Consider referral to a psychiatric care provider, if indicated
- Consider short-term psychotherapy and/or psychopharmacology

---

10–14 days after delivery

- Likely transient depression ("postpartum blues")[2]
- Exclude postpartum psychosis[3]

Inpatient management of psychosis[4]

- Admit to acute psychiatric inpatient unit
- Initiate antipsychotic medications
- *Consider ECT, if indicated*

Discharge once stabilized

- Supportive care
- Monthly follow-up
- Continue breastfeeding[5]

2–3 months after delivery

- Likely postpartum depression[6]

Outpatient management

- Supportive care
- Monthly follow-up
- Continue breastfeeding[5]

Good response

- Continue supportive care and regular follow-up

Poor response

- Consider referral to a psychiatric care provider, if indicated
- Consider short-term psychotherapy and/or psychopharmacology

Obstetric Clinical Algorithms: Management and Evidence. By © E.R. Norwitz, M. Belfort, G.R. Saade and H. Miller.
Published 2010 Blackwell Publishing.

1. Pregnancy is generally thought of as a time of universal well-being. However, in women with established psychiatric disorders, pregnancy may exacerbate their symptoms. A patient's underlying psychiatric diagnosis as well as her social, cultural, and educational background will often determine her emotional adjustment to being pregnant. In general, pregnancies that are planned and/or desired create fewer conflicts within the individual and as such are better accepted. The puerperium has long been identified as a time of increased risk for mental illness. This is due in part to discontinuation of medications during pregnancy because of concern over the safety of the fetus.

2. A mild transient depression ("postpartum blues" or "maternity blues") is common immediately after delivery, occurring in >50% of all postpartum women. The etiology of this disorder is unclear, but is likely due to the rapid biochemical and hormonal changes associated with childbirth.

3. Severe postpartum psychotic depressive or manic illness is rare (1–2 per 1000 livebirths). Risk factors include younger age, primiparity, a family history of mental illness, and most especially a personal history of psychotic illness. The risk of recurrence in a woman with a history of postpartum psychosis is 25–30%. The peak onset of psychotic symptoms is typically 10–14 days after delivery.

4. In patients with postpartum psychosis, pharmacologic therapy should be initiated as soon as possible and short-term hospitalization may be necessary. Electroconvulsant therapy (ECT) has been used in this setting with some success. Many of these women go on to develop life-long depressive disorders. Interestingly, suicide is uncommon during pregnancy and the year following delivery. Recurrence of postpartum psychosis is high (25–30%)

5. All psychotropic drugs are excreted in breast milk. The milk-to-plasma ratio of antidepressants ranges from 0.5 to 1.0, whereas only 40% of lithium is excreted in breast milk. In general, the amount of medication ingested by the baby is small. For this reason, the American Academy of Pediatrics (1983) has concluded that antipsychotic drugs and lithium are compatible with breastfeeding. However, metabolism of drugs is impaired in infants due to hepatic immaturity. This is especially true for premature infants, and in this cohort it may be prudent to withhold breast milk if high doses of medication are required. An alternative recommendation has been to continue breastfeeding, but to monitor maternal and infant blood levels and discontinue feeding only if the drug levels are dangerously elevated or if the infant develops sign of toxicity.

6. Nonpsychotic postpartum depression complicates approximately 8–15% of all pregnancies, but the incidence may be as high as 30% in women with a prior history of depression and upwards of 70–85% in women with a previous episode of postpartum depression. Symptoms typically start between 2 and 3 months after delivery.

7. Prophylactic pharmacotherapy should be considered in such cases. Unfortunately, depressive illness is only identified in around one-third to one-half of postpartum patients who meet *Diagnostic and statistical manual (DSM)-IV* diagnostic criteria. The natural history of a postpartum depressive episode is one of gradual improvement over the 6–12 months following delivery. Supportive care and monthly follow-up for the first 3–6 months (watching for symptoms and signs of worsening depression, thoughts of infanticide or suicide, emergence of psychosis, and response to treatment) may be all that is required.

69 Sterilization[1]

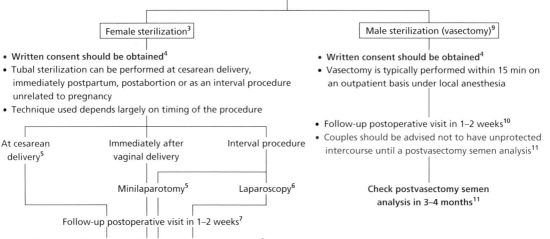

Couple requesting sterilization

- Couples requesting sterilization should be counseled about the nature, efficacy, safety, and complications of the various surgical procedures
- Couples should be made aware of all available alternative methods of contraception
- Couples should understand that such procedures are intended to be permanent[2]

Female sterilization[3]

- Written consent should be obtained[4]
- Tubal sterilization can be performed at cesarean delivery, immediately postpartum, postabortion or as an interval procedure unrelated to pregnancy
- Technique used depends largely on timing of the procedure

At cesarean delivery[5]

Immediately after vaginal delivery

Interval procedure

Minilaparotomy[5]   Laparoscopy[6]

Follow-up postoperative visit in 1–2 weeks[7]

If amenorrheic, women should check a pregnancy test[8]

Male sterilization (vasectomy)[9]

- Written consent should be obtained[4]
- Vasectomy is typically performed within 15 min on an outpatient basis under local anesthesia

- Follow-up postoperative visit in 1–2 weeks[10]
- Couples should be advised not to have unprotected intercourse until a postvasectomy semen analysis[11]

Check postvasectomy semen analysis in 3–4 months[11]

Obstetric Clinical Algorithms: Management and Evidence. By © E.R. Norwitz, M. Belfort, G.R. Saade and H. Miller.
Published 2010 Blackwell Publishing.

1. Sterilization refers to a surgical procedure that is aimed at permanently blocking or removing part of the female or male genital tract to prevent fertilization. It is the most common method of family planning worldwide. Over 175 million couples use surgical sterilization for contraception, 90% of whom live in developing countries. The ratio of female to male sterilization is 3:1.

2. Sterilization is designed to be permanent. That said, microsurgical tubal reanastomosis has good results if a small segment of the tube has been damaged. As such, pregnancy rates following reanastomosis are low with electrocoagulation and higher with clips, rings, and surgical methods. Vas deferens reanastomosis is a difficult and meticulous surgical procedure that has only a 50% success rate. The strongest indicator of future regret is young age at the time of sterilization, regardless of parity or marital status. Consider obtaining a social service consult if the patient is young or has few children.

3. Female sterilization refers to permanent surgical interruption of the fallopian tubes bilaterally. The procedure is immediately effective.

4. State laws and/or insurance regulations often require a specific interval between obtaining consent and surgical sterilization.

5. The minilaparotomy approach can be used in the interval, postabortion or postpartum period. Interval minilaparotomy is performed through a 2–3 cm midline suprapubic incision. The abdomen is entered, the uterus is identified, and a finger is used to elevate the fallopian tube. After the tube has been identified by its fimbriated end, the mid-portion is grasped with a Babcock clamp. Tubal occlusion is then performed. If a segment of tube is removed, it should be sent to pathology to confirm a complete cross-section of fallopian tube. A similar procedure can be carried out following vaginal delivery (postpartum sterilization – PPS). The latter procedure is ideally performed while the uterine fundus is high in the abdomen (typically within 48 hours of delivery). Maternal and neonatal well-being should be confirmed prior to PPS.

6. Laparoscopic tubal ligation (LTL) is performed using one or more trocar instruments in addition to the umbilical camera site. Advantages of the laparoscopic approach over other surgical procedures include the opportunity to inspect the abdominal and pelvic organs, small incision scars, and a more rapid postoperative recovery. Techniques of tubal occlusion include the following.

- *Electrocoagulation*: bipolar cautery is safer than unipolar cautery, which has the potential to cause thermal bowel injury.
- *Clips and rings*: mechanical occlusion devices, such as the silicone rubber band (Falope ring) and the spring-loaded clip (Hulka clip, Filshie clip), are less commonly used for LTL. Special applicators are necessary and each requires skill for proper application. Clips and rings destroy less oviductal tissue than electrocoagulation. Tubal adhesions or a thickened or dilated fallopian tube increase the risk of misapplication of the clip.

7. Complications of tubal ligation are rare. The mortality rate (1–2 per 100,000 procedures in the United States) is lower than that for childbirth (10 per 100,000 births). Anesthetic complication is the leading cause of death. Other potential complications include hemorrhage, infection, erroneous ligation of the round ligament, and injury to adjacent structures. Overall, when the risk of pregnancy from contraceptive failure is taken into account, sterilization is the safest of all contraceptive methods.

8. The failure rate of tubal ligation is dependent upon the specific operation, the skill of the operator, and characteristics of the patient (age, pelvic adhesions, hydrosalpinx). When sterilization failure occurs, the resultant pregnancy is more likely to be an ectopic (tubal) pregnancy.

9. Vasectomy involves permanent surgical interruption of the vas deferens (the duct that transports sperm during ejaculation) bilaterally. Pregnancy rates following vasectomy are <1%. When compared with female tubal sterilization, vasectomy is safer, less expensive, and equally effective.

10. Postoperative complications of vasectomy include wound hematomas, infections, and rarely sperm granulomas (<3%). Putative long-term side-effects (increased risk of prostate cancer, decreased libido) have never been proven.

11. Unlike tubal occlusion in women, vasectomy is not immediately effective. Spermatozoa normally mature in the vas deferens for around 70 days prior to ejaculation. For this reason, 3 months or 20 ejaculations are needed to completely deplete the vas deferens of viable sperm. Postvasectomy semen analysis should be performed to determine the effectiveness of the procedure prior to unprotected intercourse.

SECTION 6
Obstetric Emergencies

70 Acute Abdomen in Pregnancy

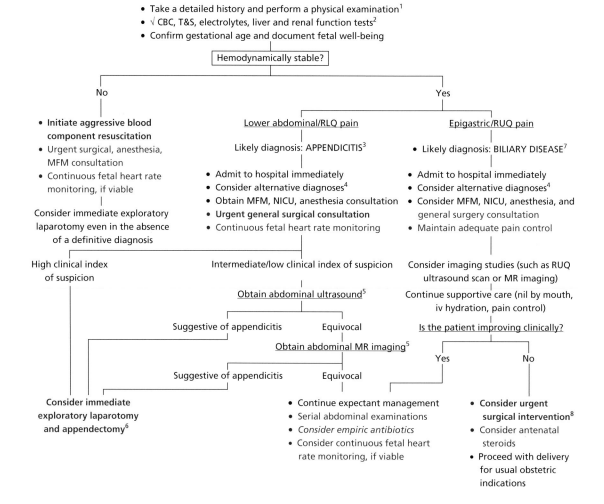

- Take a detailed history and perform a physical examination[1]
- √ CBC, T&S, electrolytes, liver and renal function tests[2]
- Confirm gestational age and document fetal well-being

Hemodynamically stable?

No

- **Initiate aggressive blood component resuscitation**
- Urgent surgical, anesthesia, MFM consultation
- Continuous fetal heart rate monitoring, if viable

Consider immediate exploratory laparotomy even in the absence of a definitive diagnosis

High clinical index of suspicion

Consider immediate exploratory laparotomy and appendectomy[6]

Yes

Lower abdominal/RLQ pain

Likely diagnosis: APPENDICITIS[3]

- Admit to hospital immediately
- Consider alternative diagnoses[4]
- Obtain MFM, NICU, anesthesia consultation
- **Urgent general surgical consultation**
- Continuous fetal heart rate monitoring

Intermediate/low clinical index of suspicion

Obtain abdominal ultrasound[5]

Suggestive of appendicitis   Equivocal

Obtain abdominal MR imaging[5]

Suggestive of appendicitis   Equivocal

- Continue expectant management
- Serial abdominal examinations
- *Consider empiric antibiotics*
- Consider continuous fetal heart rate monitoring, if viable

Epigastric/RUQ pain

- Likely diagnosis: BILIARY DISEASE[7]

- Admit to hospital immediately
- Consider alternative diagnoses[4]
- Consider MFM, NICU, anesthesia, and general surgery consultation
- Maintain adequate pain control

Consider imaging studies (such as RUQ ultrasound scan or MR imaging)

Continue supportive care (nil by mouth, iv hydration, pain control)

Is the patient improving clinically?

Yes   No

- **Consider urgent surgical intervention[8]**
- Consider antenatal steroids
- Proceed with delivery for usual obstetric indications

Obstetric Clinical Algorithms: Management and Evidence. By © E.R. Norwitz, M. Belfort, G.R. Saade and H. Miller.
Published 2010 Blackwell Publishing.

1. History should be brief and focused. Ask about underlying medical conditions, prior surgery, medications and allergies. Ask about pregnancy complications including vaginal bleeding, leakage of fluid, contractions, and fetal movements. Physical examination may reveal generalized or focal tenderness, presence/absence of guarding and rebound tenderness, and increased/decreased bowel sounds. Confirm gestational age and document fetal well-being, especially if >24 weeks' gestation.

2. White blood cell count in normal pregnancy ranges from 6000 to 16,000 cell/mm^3 but counts that are significantly higher than that or have evidence of a left shift suggest underlying infection/inflammation.

3. Acute appendicitis is the most common general surgical problem encountered during pregnancy, complicating 1 in 1500 deliveries. It is not more common in pregnancy, but pregnancy is associated with a higher rate of perforation likely due to delay in diagnosis. The clinical manifestations and diagnosis of appendicitis in pregnancy are similar to those in nonpregnant individuals (abdominal pain, fever, gastrointestinal upset, elevated WCC) with a few exceptions: (i) RLQ pain is commonly reported, but the point of maximal tenderness may be higher than McBurney's point because of the upward displacement of the appendix with increasing gestational age; (ii) indigestion, anorexia, bowel irregularity, nausea/vomiting, and a sense of not feeling well are common symptoms, but may be confused with normal pregnancy. Nausea and vomiting following the onset of abdominal pain suggests appendicitis.

4. The differential diagnosis is extensive, including any cause of abdominal pain including, among others, gastroenteritis, constipation, peptic ulcer disease, small bowel obstruction, inflammatory bowel disease (Crohn disease or ulcerative colitis), pancreatitis, ectopic pregnancy, ruptured ovarian cyst, ovarian torsion, renal colic, pyelonephritis, and (rarely) such disorders as sickle cell crisis, pneumonia, diabetic ketoacidosis, porphyria.

5. Abdominal ultrasonography is recommended in pregnant patients suspected of having appendicitis. If ultrasonography suggests appendicitis, surgery is indicated.

If clinical findings and ultrasound are inconclusive, magnetic resonance (MR) imaging should be considered, where available, because it avoids fetal exposure to ionizing radiation and performs well in diagnosis of lower abdominal/pelvic disorders. If MR imaging suggests appendicitis, surgery is indicated. Computed tomography (CT) imaging can be used when MR imaging is not available, given its proven value in nonpregnant individuals.

6. The decision to proceed to laparotomy should be based upon the clinical findings, diagnostic imaging results, and clinical judgment. Laboratory tests are not particularly useful other than to rule in an alternative diagnosis. Delaying intervention for more than 24 hours increases the risk of perforation. When the diagnosis is relatively certain, appendectomy can be performed through a transverse incision over the point of maximal tenderness. However, when the diagnosis is less certain or if there is a chance that a cesarean delivery may need to be performed (for example, in the setting of early labor), it may be more prudent to approach the appendix through a lower midline vertical or paramedian incision.

7. The incidence of biliary disease (biliary colic, cholecystitis) requiring surgery is one case per 2000 pregnancies. Hormonal changes associated with pregnancy predispose to the development of gallstones (cholelithiasis) by increasing the viscosity of bile, increasing the number of micelles on which cholesterol crystals precipitate, and relaxing the gallbladder, leading to stasis. Cholelithiasis is the main cause of cholecystitis in pregnancy, accounting for >90% of cases.

8. Many patients will improve with supportive care; those who continue to have severe symptoms and show no improvement despite medical management require further intervention. If gangrene or perforation is suspected either clinically or on imaging studies or if there are signs of instability (progressive fever, intractable pain) while on supportive therapy, urgent surgical intervention must be considered to remove the offending inflamed, gangrenous or perforated gallbladder. A laparoscopic approach may be possible prior to 30 weeks' gestation.

71 Acute Asthma Exacerbation

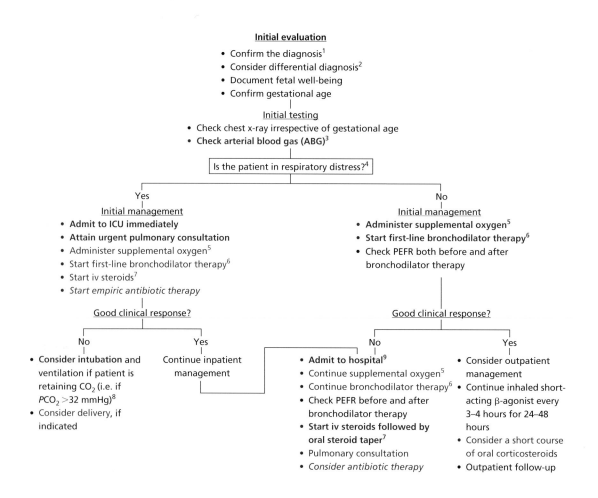

Initial evaluation

- Confirm the diagnosis[1]
- Consider differential diagnosis[2]
- Document fetal well-being
- Confirm gestational age

Initial testing
- Check chest x-ray irrespective of gestational age
- Check arterial blood gas (ABG)[3]

Is the patient in respiratory distress?[4]

Yes

Initial management
- **Admit to ICU immediately**
- **Attain urgent pulmonary consultation**
- Administer supplemental oxygen[5]
- Start first-line bronchodilator therapy[6]
- Start iv steroids[7]
- *Start empiric antibiotic therapy*

Good clinical response?

No
- **Consider intubation and ventilation if patient is retaining CO2** (i.e. if $PCO_2 >32$ mmHg)[8]
- Consider delivery, if indicated

Yes
Continue inpatient management

No

Initial management
- **Administer supplemental oxygen[5]**
- **Start first-line bronchodilator therapy[6]**
- Check PEFR both before and after bronchodilator therapy

Good clinical response?

No
- **Admit to hospital[9]**
- Continue supplemental oxygen[5]
- Continue bronchodilator therapy[6]
- Check PEFR before and after bronchodilator therapy
- **Start iv steroids followed by oral steroid taper[7]**
- Pulmonary consultation
- *Consider antibiotic therapy*

Yes
- Consider outpatient management
- Continue inhaled short-acting β-agonist every 3–4 hours for 24–48 hours
- Consider a short course of oral corticosteroids
- Outpatient follow-up

Obstetric Clinical Algorithms: Management and Evidence. By © E.R. Norwitz, M. Belfort, G.R. Saade and H. Miller.
Published 2010 Blackwell Publishing.

1. Asthma is a chronic inflammatory disorder of the airways characterized by intermittent episodes of reversible bronchospasm. The "classic" signs and symptoms of asthma are intermittent dyspnea, cough, and wheezing. To confirm the diagnosis, take a detailed history, perform a physical examination, and perform relevant pulmonary function tests, including peak expiratory flow rate (PEFR) and spirometry, which includes measurement of forced expiratory volume in 1 second (FEV1) and forced vital capacity (FVC) before and after administration of a bronchodilator.

2. The differential diagnosis of an acute asthma exacerbation includes pneumonia, pulmonary embolism, pneumothorax, congestive cardiac failure, pericarditis, pulmonary edema, and rib fracture.

3. Respiratory adaptations in pregnancy are designed to optimize maternal and fetal oxygenation, and to facilitate transfer of CO_2 waste from the fetus to the mother (see Chapter 6). Pregnancy thus represents a state of *compensated respiratory alkalosis.*

	pH	Po_2 (mmHg)	Pco_2 (mmHg)
Nonpregnant	7.40	93–100	35–40
Pregnant	7.40	100–105	28–30

4. Symptoms and signs suggestive of a serious asthma attack and respiratory distress include marked breathlessness, inability to speak more than short phrases, use of accessory muscles or drowsiness. A PEFR of <40% expected or of personal best (or <200 L/min in most adults) indicates a need for urgent medical intervention.

5. Supplemental oxygen is typically administered by nonrebreather mask at 4-8 L/min to keep the O_2 saturation >95% in pregnancy (>92% in nonpregnant women).

6. As initial treatment, inhaled short-acting β-agonists should be used early and frequently. Albuterol can be given either as 4–8 puffs of a metered dose inhaler (MDI) with spacer every 20 minutes for up to 4 hours or by nebulizer treatment (2.5 mg repeated every 20 minutes for two or three doses or 10–15 mg given by continuous nebulization over 1 hour). Consider concomitant use of ipratropium bromide for severe exacerbations given as 500 g by nebulization every 20 minutes for three doses or eight puffs by MDI with spacer every 20 minutes as needed for up to 3 hours.

7. Start systemic glucocorticoids if there is not an immediate and marked response to the inhaled short-acting β-agonists. Recommended steroid regimens include methylprednisolone 60–125 mg iv or prednisone 40–60 mg orally; alternative regimens include dexametasone 6–10 mg iv or hydrocortisone 150–200 mg iv. Steroids may be given im or orally if iv access is unavailable. Steroids should be repeated at 8–12 hour intervals. Other treatment options for asthma that is severe and unresponsive to standard therapies include terbutaline (0.25 mg by sc injection every 30 minutes for three doses) or epinephrine (0.2–0.5 mL of 1:1000 solution by sc injection). Give terbutaline or epinephrine, but not both.

8. Hypercapnia (a sign of impending respiratory failure) usually only occurs if the PEFR is <25% of normal (or <100–150 L/min). If intubation difficulty is not anticipated, rapid sequence intubation is preferred. Nasal intubation is not recommended.

9. Patients should be admitted to hospital if they do not respond well after 4–6 hours in a setting of high surveillance and care. Frequent (every 1–2 hours) objective clinical assessments of the response to therapy are needed once admitted until a definite and sustained improvement is documented.

72 Acute Shortness of Breath

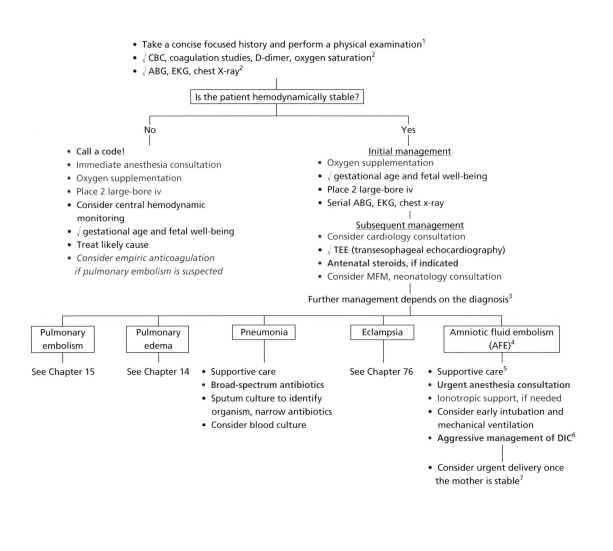

- Take a concise focused history and perform a physical examination[1]
- √ CBC, coagulation studies, D-dimer, oxygen saturation[2]
- √ ABG, EKG, chest X-ray[2]

Is the patient hemodynamically stable?

No

- **Call a code!**
- Immediate anesthesia consultation
- Oxygen supplementation
- Place 2 large-bore iv
- **Consider central hemodynamic monitoring**
- √ gestational age and fetal well-being
- **Treat likely cause**
- *Consider empiric anticoagulation if pulmonary embolism is suspected*

Yes

Initial management
- Oxygen supplementation
- √ gestational age and fetal well-being
- Place 2 large-bore iv
- Serial ABG, EKG, chest x-ray

Subsequent management
- Consider cardiology consultation
- √ TEE (transesophageal echocardiography)
- **Antenatal steroids, if indicated**
- Consider MFM, neonatology consultation

Further management depends on the diagnosis[3]

Pulmonary embolism

See Chapter 15

Pulmonary edema

See Chapter 14

Pneumonia

- Supportive care
- **Broad-spectrum antibiotics**
- Sputum culture to identify organism, narrow antibiotics
- Consider blood culture

Eclampsia

See Chapter 76

Amniotic fluid embolism (AFE)[4]

- Supportive care[5]
- **Urgent anesthesia consultation**
- Ionotropic support, if needed
- Consider early intubation and mechanical ventilation
- **Aggressive management of DIC[6]**

- **Consider urgent delivery once the mother is stable[7]**

Obstetric Clinical Algorithms: Management and Evidence. By © E.R. Norwitz, M. Belfort, G.R. Saade and H. Miller.
Published 2010 Blackwell Publishing.

1. Ask about acute-onset shortness of breath (dyspnea), pleuritic chest pain, cough, and/or hemoptysis. On examination, look for low-grade fever, tachypnea, tachycardia, diminished oxygen saturation, diminished breath sounds, audible crackles, and/or evidence of pleural effusion on pulmonary examination.

2. Laboratory tests may reveal acidosis and an elevated A-a gradient on arterial blood gas analysis (ABG), and evidence of right heart strain (S1Q3T3 pattern with or without right axis deviation, T wave inversion) on EKG. CXR may be normal or show evidence of multiple peripheral wedge-shaped areas of consolidation, pulmonary edema, and/or pleural effusion. However, if ABG reveals an arterial $pO_2 > 80$ mmHg, the diagnosis of PE is highly unlikely. Similarly, although D-dimer levels are not generally helpful in making the diagnosis of PE, a clinically significant VTE is highly unlikely if the D-dimer is normal.

3. The differential diagnosis of acute shortness of breath includes pulmonary embolism, amniotic fluid embolism, pneumonia (including aspiration pneumonitis – Mendelson syndrome), pneumothorax, congestive cardiac failure, pericarditis, pulmonary edema, venous air embolism (rare, associated with ruptured uterus, placenta previa, and persistent atrial septal defect), eclampsia, drug overdose/withdrawal, and rib fracture.

4. *Amniotic fluid embolism* (AFE) is an obstetric emergency with 80–90% maternal and perinatal mortality. It accounts for 10% of maternal deaths in the US. AFE is seen most commonly during labor and delivery, and in the immediate postpartum period. Risk factors include cesarean delivery, chorioamnionitis, multiparity, pre-eclampsia, prolonged labor, fetal demise, "excessive" oxytocin augmentation, amniotomy, intrauterine pressure catheter, intrauterine saline injection (abortion), and placental abruption. It is characterized by acute-onset dyspnea, hypotension, and hypoxemia. Prodromal symptoms may include sudden chills, sweating or anxiety. Physical examination may reveal acute-onset respiratory distress, cyanosis, hypotension, tachycardia, hypoxemia, neurologic manifestations (seizures, coma), and/or hemorrhage. AFE is a clinical diagnosis. CXR and V/Q scan are of little value in the acute setting. Components of amniotic fluid (fetal squames, mucin) may be identified in the pulmonary vasculature at postmortem, but are not pathognomonic.

5. Therapy is primarily supportive. Cardiovascular support should be optimized. This includes maintaining O_2 saturation >90%, arterial PO_2 >60 mmHg, systolic BP >90 mmHg, and urine output >25 mL/h. Ionotropic support (dopamine) and mechanical ventilation should be considered, if needed. Treat bronchospasm (terbutaline, aminophylline, steroids) as needed. CPR and cardiopulmonary bypass may be required.

6. Disseminated intravascular coagulopathy (DIC) is typically a predominant clinical feature of AFE. Serial CBC and coagulation studies should be followed, and aggressive blood product replacement initiated. Avoid heparin in established DIC.

7. The fetus is at risk of hypoxic ischemic cerebral injury and/or IUFD. Urgent delivery may be necessary regardless of gestational age. Regional anesthesia is contraindicated in the acute setting. General endotracheal anesthesia may be needed for cesarean.

73 Cord Prolapse

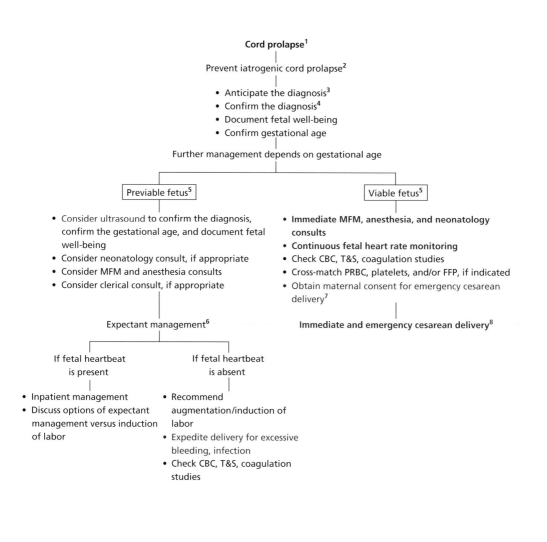

Cord prolapse[1]
|
Prevent iatrogenic cord prolapse[2]
|
- Anticipate the diagnosis[3]
- Confirm the diagnosis[4]
- Document fetal well-being
- Confirm gestational age
|
Further management depends on gestational age

Previable fetus[5]

- Consider ultrasound to confirm the diagnosis, confirm the gestational age, and document fetal well-being
- Consider neonatology consult, if appropriate
- Consider MFM and anesthesia consults
- Consider clerical consult, if appropriate

Expectant management[6]

If fetal heartbeat is present
- Inpatient management
- Discuss options of expectant management versus induction of labor

If fetal heartbeat is absent
- Recommend augmentation/induction of labor
- Expedite delivery for excessive bleeding, infection
- Check CBC, T&S, coagulation studies

Viable fetus[5]

- **Immediate MFM, anesthesia, and neonatology consults**
- **Continuous fetal heart rate monitoring**
- Check CBC, T&S, coagulation studies
- Cross-match PRBC, platelets, and/or FFP, if indicated
- Obtain maternal consent for emergency cesarean delivery[7]

Immediate and emergency cesarean delivery[8]

Obstetric Clinical Algorithms: Management and Evidence. By © E.R. Norwitz, M. Belfort, G.R. Saade and H. Miller.
Published 2010 Blackwell Publishing.

1. Cord prolapse is an obstetric emergency characterized by prolapse of the umbilical cord into the vagina after rupture of the fetal membranes.

2. To prevent iatrogenic cord prolapse, perform amniotomy (artificial rupture of the membranes) only once the vertex is well applied to the cervix and always with fundal pressure.

3. The diagnosis should be anticipated in the setting of rupture of the fetal membranes if any of the following risk factors are present: (i) prematurity; (ii) a small fetus; (iii) funic presentation on prior ultrasound examination; and (iv) fetal malpresentation (Incidence at term is 0.4% of cephalic pregnancies, 0.5% of frank breech pregnancies, 4–6% of complete breech pregnancies, 15–18% of footling breech pregnancies, and may be >25% with transverse lie.

4. Cord prolapse is a *clinical* diagnosis made by palpation of the pulsatile cord on vaginal examination with or without fetal bradycardia. In the acute setting with a viable fetus, there is no place for ultrasound to confirm the diagnosis.

5. Fetal viability is variably defined. In the US, most obstetric care providers would currently regard the limit of fetal viability as being between 23 and 24 weeks of gestation.

6. Contraindications to expectant management include intrauterine fetal demise, infection, hemodynamic instability (shock), excessive bleeding, and coagulopathy.

7. Given the urgency of the situation, verbal consent for surgery is likely adequate. However, the obstetric care provider may want to consider getting a witness to document verbal consent and getting written consent from the patient once she has fully recovered from anesthesia. If this is done, it should be made clear that the written consent was obtained after the procedure.

8. Once the diagnosis of cord prolapse has been made in a viable pregnancy with confirmation of a live fetus (usually by palpation of a pulsatile cord), the management should include the following.
- CALL FOR HELP.
- Manual replacement of the umbilical cord into the uterus by the obstetric care provider, who should continue manual replacement until the infant is delivered.
- Place the patient in the knee–chest position.
- Establish intravenous access.
- O_2 supplementation by facemask.
- Transfer the patient immediately to the operating room.
- Immediate anesthesia, neonatology, and/or obstetric consult, if indicated.
- Check emergency CBC, T&S, coagulation studies.
- Continued assessment of fetal well-being (usually confirmation of a pulsatile umbilical cord is adequate).
- Emergency cesarean delivery, usually under general endotracheal anesthesia (epidural analgesia may be used only if it is already in place and has been tested).

74 Cardiopulmonary Resuscitation

<u>CPR in pregnancy</u>[1]

- Be aware of the physiologic changes in pregnancy which may predispose to acute cardiovascular collapse[2]
- Understand risk factors for cardiovascular collapse[3]

| Confirm acute cardiovascular collapse |

<u>Initial interventions</u>

- **Call for help. Call a code!**
- **A – Airway** (turn patient on her side, ensure airway is patent, consider early intubation)
- **B – Breathing** (ensure patient is breathing; if not, perform chest compressions/CPR while preparing for intubation and ventilation)
- **C – Circulation** (place 2 large-bore iv, initiate fluid resuscitation, order blood products)

<u>Subsequent management</u>

- √ **CBC, liver/renal function tests, coagulation profile**
- √ **EKG, arterial blood gas, CXR, toxicology screen**
- Initiate rule out myocardial infarction protocol
- Consider differential diagnosis and manage accordingly[3]
- **Continue aggressive CPR, including early intubation and left lateral tilt[4]**

| Initial resuscitation efforts successful |

- Transfer to ICU
- Confirm gestational age and fetal well-being[5]
- Search for an underlying cause

| Resuscitation unsuccessful |

Confirm gestational age and fetal well-being[5]

Gestational age <24 weeks and/or nonviable fetus

- **Continue aggressive CPR**
- Consider emptying the uterus within 5–10 min to facilitate CPR[6]
- Transfer to ICU once stable
- Continue to search for an underlying cause

Gestational age ≥24 weeks and a viable fetus

- **Empty the uterus within 5–10 min[6]**
- Pediatrics present at delivery
- Continue aggressive CPR
- Transfer to ICU once stable
- Continue to search for an underlying cause

Obstetric Clinical Algorithms: Management and Evidence. By © E.R. Norwitz, M. Belfort, G.R. Saade and H. Miller.
Published 2010 Blackwell Publishing.

1. Cardiovascular collapse may occur in pregnancy as it does in nonpregnant women. Obstetricians should be able to anticipate, diagnose, and manage acute cardiovascular collapse. Being an obstetric care provider is no excuse for being CPR illiterate.

2. Physiologic adaptations in the mother occur in response to the demands of pregnancy, which include: (i) support of the fetus (volume, nutritional and oxygen support, clearance of fetal waste); (ii) protection of the fetus from starvation, drugs, and toxins; (iii) preparation of the uterus for labor; and (iv) protection of the mother from potential cardiovascular injury at delivery. All maternal organ systems are required to adapt to the demands of pregnancy. Most importantly, pregnancy is a state of increased metabolic demand and yet the buffering capacity of the body is diminished in pregnancy. The placenta serves as a low-resistance, high-capacity shunt which accommodates 20–30% of the cardiac output at term, but lacks autonomic innervation and, as such, is unable to shut down in the setting of hypovolemia. Pregnancy is associated with a dilutional anemia and a reduction in functional residual capacity, both of which limit the ability of a pregnant woman to meet the demands of acute cardiovascular collapse. Moreover, significant aortocaval compression occurs after 20 weeks' gestation due to the rapidly enlarging uterus, which may significantly reduce the effectiveness of CPR. Pregnant women are also at increased risk of aspiration chemical pneumonitis (Mendelson syndrome).

3. Acute cardiovascular collapse in pregnancy typically occurs in the setting of one or more predisposing conditions. These include massive blood loss (either concealed or revealed hemorrhage), sepsis, pulmonary embolism, amniotic fluid embolism, pre-eclampsia, and coagulopathy. Management should be tailored to the likely cause. For example, empiric broad-spectrum antibiotics should be started immediately if septic shock is suspected. If massive blood loss is suspected, the source of the blood loss should be identified and stopped, fluid resuscitation should be started, and coagulopathy aggressively treated

4. Early intubation and ventilation has been associated with improved outcome for both mother and fetus. Although a number of acute interventions have not been well studied in pregnancy, few interventions are absolutely contraindicated when the alternative is death. These interventions include many inotrope and vasopressor medications (which will likely reduce uteroplacental blood flow) and thrombolytics (for the acute management of myocardial infarction and pulmonary embolism). If a cardiac dysrhythmia is suspected or develops as a result of the cardiovascular collapse, consider immediate defibrillation (shock).

5. Initial efforts at maternal resuscitation should not be delayed to document fetal well-being.

6. Cardiopulmonary resuscitation does not adequately perfuse the uterus, and neonatal neurologic impairment increases significantly after 8–10 minutes of CPR. Moreover, uterine size> 20 weeks has been associated with significant aortocaval compression which will interfere with CPR. As such, if CPR has not been successful within 5–10 minutes, both maternal resuscitative efforts and intact fetal salvage will be improved if the uterus is immediately evacuated (so-called perimortem cesarean delivery). In this emergency setting, patient consent is not required. A vertical skin incision should be performed followed by a high vertical ("classic") hysterotomy. The uterine content should be evaluated immediately. If the fetus is viable, it should be passed off to the waiting pediatricians. Adequate maternal analgesia is essential, and this can be rapidly achieved though general anesthesia since the patient is typically intubated. The uterus should be rapidly closed using a single full-thickness suture. The abdomen should be left open (covered with a sterile transparent sheet) to ensure that the uterus does not fill with blood, thereby further impairing CPR. The skin can be closed at a later time. CPR should be continued throughout this procedure.

75 Diabetic Ketoacidosis[1]

- Identify women at risk of developing DKA[2]
- Education to prevent DKA[3]

Confirm the diagnosis[4]

- Perform a detailed history and physical examination
- Send the following diagnostic tests: glucose, CBC, electrolytes, arterial blood gas (ABG), urinalysis, and serum and urinary ketones

Unable to confirm the diagnosis[5]

- Consider other diagnoses[6]
- Confirm gestational age
- Document fetal well-being

Manage as an outpatient and continue strict glycemic control

Diagnosis of DKA is confirmed[5]

- Admit to hospital
- Confirm gestational age
- Document fetal well-being
- Exclude infection as a cause of DKA: check blood cultures, urine culture, and a CXR if indicated

Institute treatment immediately[7]

- **Manage in ICU setting** with q 15 min maternal vital signs, EKG, facemask oxygen supplementation at 4–6 L/min
- Continuous fetal monitoring if >24 weeks' gestation

Treat hyperglycemia

- **10 units regular insulin iv push** followed by infusion of 6 units per hour (0.1 units/kg per hour) in NS[8]
- Check serum glucose hourly
- Aim to decrease serum glucose by 60 mg/dL each hour
- Stop insulin for 1 hour if serum glucose <80 mg/dL

Treat volume deficit

- Average water deficit is 10% of total bodyweight
- **Replace half of the 4–5 L fluid deficit within the first 5 hours** (~1 L per hour)
- Give NS; change to ½NS if sodium >155 mEq/L; add 5% dextrose once serum glucose <250 mg/dL

Treat electrolyte imbalance

- Add 10–40 mEq KCl per liter of iv fluid
- Check serum potassium levels hourly
- Maintain potassium levels at 4–5 mEq/L
- Stop KCl infusion if levels are >5.5 mEq/L or if there is oliguria

Treat acidosis

- *If pH <7.0, consider bicarbonate* (2 amps [88 mEq] $NaHCO_3$ in 100 mL NS given iv over 45–60 min)
- Check acid–base status every 30 min if the pH remains <7.0[9]

Treat infection

- *Consider administering broad-spectrum iv antibiotics,* if underlying infection is suspected as the cause of DKA

Once the patient is stable, continue close observation[10]

Obstetric Clinical Algorithms: Management and Evidence. By © E.R. Norwitz, M. Belfort, G.R. Saade and H. Miller.
Published 2010 Blackwell Publishing.

1. Diabetic ketoacidosis (DKA) results from a relative or absolute deficiency of circulating insulin in the setting of excessive glucose counter-regulatory hormones (catecholamines, growth hormone, cortisol, and glucagon). Insulin is an anabolic hormone that drives glucose into cells. Insulin deficiency results in a fundamental paradox: although there is an adequate supply of glucose, the body believes that it is starving and begins to make ketones for use by the vital organs (heart and brain). This leads to ketoacidosis in the setting of hyperglycemia.

2. Diabetic ketoacidosis develops in 2–10% of all pregnancies complicated by pregestational diabetes. It is extremely rare in gestational diabetes ($\ll$1%), and effectively absent in nondiabetic women. Risk factors for the development of DKA include undiagnosed pregestational diabetes, pregnancy, emesis, noncompliance, infection, β-agonist therapy, and (perhaps) antepartum corticosteroid therapy.

3. Diabetic ketoacidosis can be effectively prevented by intensive diabetic education, rigorous glycemic control, and early identification and treatment of infection.

4. A high clinical index of suspicion is necessary to make the diagnosis of DKA. Any pregnant women with pregestational diabetes who complains of nausea, vomiting, polydipsia, polyuria, abdominal pain, and/or decreased caloric intake should be evaluated to exclude ketosis. Physical examination may demonstrate dehydration, poor tissue turgor, tachycardia, hypotension, a fruity smell (acetone) on breath, and clinical evidence of acidosis (fatigue, hyperventilation and Kussmaul breathing or coma).

5. The following five criteria are typically used for the diagnosis of DKA.
- Plasma glucose >250 mg/dL (although normal or near-normal plasma glucose levels are not sufficient to preclude DKA; indeed, up to 40% of pregnant diabetic women with DKA have plasma glucose levels on presentation of <200 mg/dL)
- pH <7.30
- Plasma bicarbonate <15 mEq/L
- Anion gap ($Na^+ - [Cl^- + HCO_3-]$) 12 mEq/L
- Osmolality (2 [$\times$] [$Na^+ + K^+$] + [glucose/18]) >280 mOsm/kg

6. The differential diagnosis of altered mental status in the setting of DKA includes hyperglycemic coma in women with pregestational diabetes, pre-eclampsia/eclampsia, seizure, drug overdose (especially alcohol), encephalopathy, uremia, infection, and psychosis.

7. Diabetic ketoacidosis is associated with a high maternal (5%) and perinatal mortality (35–50%). Other perinatal complications include preterm birth and newborn encephalopathy. Prognosis depends in large part on early diagnosis and rapid and effective inpatient treatment. The primary objectives include correction of volume deficit, hyperglycemia, electrolyte imbalance, acidosis, and treatment of the precipitating cause (infection). Babies die of acidosis and not high glucose levels. As such, the immediate goal of treatment is reversal of ketoacidosis, not euglycemia.

8. The half-life of iv insulin is 2–4 min. DKA can recur in the absence of exogenous insulin. Subcutaneous insulin should be restarted once the patient is eating.

9. If acidosis persists, consider inadequate insulin administration, sepsis or hypophosphatemia.

10. Once stable, it is important to: (i) follow fingerstick blood glucose hourly; (ii) √ serum electrolytes and ABG q 2–4 hourly, as indicated; (iii) BUN/creatinine and urinary ketones q 4 hourly; (iv) catheterize patient if unconscious or not passing urine; (v) aspirate and decompress stomach if unconscious; (vi) continuous fetal surveillance and consideration for delivery, if indicated.

76 Eclampsia

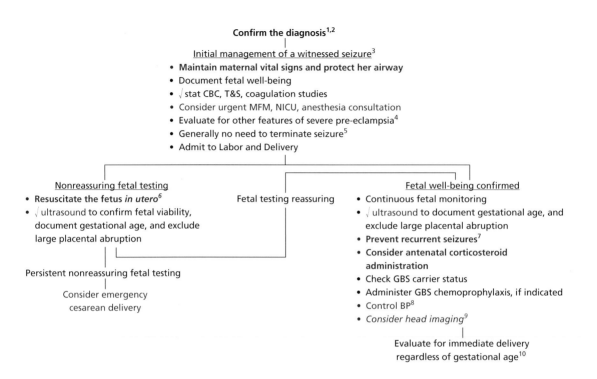

Confirm the diagnosis[1,2]

Initial management of a witnessed seizure[3]
- **Maintain maternal vital signs and protect her airway**
- Document fetal well-being
- √ stat CBC, T&S, coagulation studies
- Consider urgent MFM, NICU, anesthesia consultation
- Evaluate for other features of severe pre-eclampsia[4]
- Generally no need to terminate seizure[5]
- Admit to Labor and Delivery

Nonreassuring fetal testing
- **Resuscitate the fetus *in utero*[6]**
- √ ultrasound to confirm fetal viability, document gestational age, and exclude large placental abruption

Fetal testing reassuring

Fetal well-being confirmed
- Continuous fetal monitoring
- √ ultrasound to document gestational age, and exclude large placental abruption
- **Prevent recurrent seizures[7]**
- **Consider antenatal corticosteroid administration**
- Check GBS carrier status
- Administer GBS chemoprophylaxis, if indicated
- Control BP[8]
- *Consider head imaging[9]*

Persistent nonreassuring fetal testing

Consider emergency cesarean delivery

Evaluate for immediate delivery regardless of gestational age[10]

1. Eclampsia refers to one or more generalized convulsions and/or coma in the setting of pre-eclampsia and in the absence of other neurologic explanations. It is one manifestation of severe pre-eclampsia (see Chapter 12). Eclampsia is an obstetric emergency. Both the fetus and the mother are at immediate risk of death or life-long neurologic disability. In developed countries, the incidence of eclampsia is stable at 4–5 per 10,000 livebirths. In developing countries, the reported incidence varies from 6–7 to 100 cases per 10,000 livebirths. Eclampsia is a factor in up to 10% of all maternal deaths in developed countries.

2. Eclampsia is seen most commonly in non-white nulliparous women from lower socio-economic backgrounds. Peak incidence is in women <20 and >35 years of age; 50% of cases of eclampsia occur preterm and one-fifth occur before 31 weeks' gestation. Of those occurring at term, the majority (75%) occur either intrapartum or within 48 hours of delivery. Eclampsia can occur up to 4 weeks postpartum.

3. The immediate management of an eclamptic seizure should include maintaining maternal vital functions, controlling convulsions and blood pressure, prevention of subsequent seizures, and evaluation for delivery. If witnessed, the parturient should be rolled onto her left side and a padded tongue blade placed in her mouth to maintain airway patency and prevention of aspiration, which are the first responsibilities of management.

Obstetric Clinical Algorithms: Management and Evidence. By © E.R. Norwitz, M. Belfort, G.R. Saade and H. Miller.
Published 2010 Blackwell Publishing.

4. Other manifestations of severe pre-eclampsia may co-exist with eclampsia, including HELLP syndrome (Hemolysis, Elevated Liver enzymes and Low Platelets), disseminated intravascular coagulopathy (DIC), renal failure, hepatocellular injury, liver rupture, intracellular hemorrhage, pancreatitis, congestive cardiac failure, and pulmonary edema. This is more common in cases of eclampsia <28 weeks' gestation.

5. Eclamptic seizures are almost always self-limiting and seldom last longer than 3–4 min. As such, the administration of an agent to terminate the seizure is seldom necessary. However, if the seizure lasts >5 min, consider administering either magnesium sulfate (2–4 g iv push repeated every 15 min to a maximum of 6 g) or a benzodiazepine (such as diazepam 5–10 mg iv push repeated as required to a maximum of 50 mg) to achieve resolution.

6. Transient fetal bradycardia lasting 3–5 min is a common finding after a seizure and does not necessitate immediate delivery. Resolution of maternal seizure activity is often associated with compensatory fetal tachycardia and even with transient fetal heart rate decelerations that typically resolve within 20–30 min. Every attempt should be made to stabilize the mother and resuscitate the fetus *in utero* before making a decision about delivery.

7. Without treatment, 10% of eclamptic women will have repeated seizures. Seizure prophylaxis is thus indicated in all such women to prevent complications of recurrent seizures (neuronal death, rhabdomyolysis, metabolic acidosis, aspiration pneumonitis, pulmonary edema, and possible cerebrovascular accident). Magnesium sulfate is the prophylaxis of choice, and has been shown to be superior to diazepam, phenytoin, nimodipine, a "lytic cocktail" (promethazine hydrochloride, chlorpromazine, meperidine hydrochloride), and placebo for the prevention of repeat seizures in women with eclampsia. It is usually given as a loading dose of 4–6 g iv over 20 min followed by an infusion of 2–3 g/h. The infusion should only be given if patellar reflexes are present, respirations are >12 per min, and urine output is >100 mL in 4 hours. Although not required if the woman's clinical status is closely monitored, serum magnesium levels can be followed q6h and levels maintained at 4.8–8.4 mg/dL. Seizure prophylaxis should be continued during labor and delivery and for 24–48 hours postpartum. Exactly how magnesium acts as an anticonvulsant is not known. Possible mechanisms include selective vasodilation of the cerebral vasculature, protection of endothelial cells from damage by free radicals, prevention of calcium ion entry into ischemic cells, and/or as a competitive antagonist to the glutamate N-methyl-D-aspartate receptor (which is epileptogenic).

8. The magnitude of BP elevation is predictive of cerebrovascular accident (stroke), but not eclampsia (seizures). Antihypertensive medications should be used as needed to maintain sitting BP <160/110 mmHg to prevent stroke while effecting delivery. The antihypertensive medications of choice in this setting include hydralazine (5 mg iv push followed by 5–10 mg boluses as needed q 20 min) or labetalol (10–20 mg iv push, repeat q 10–20 min with doubling doses not to exceed 80 mg in any single dose for a maximum total cumulative dose of 300 mg).

9. Eclampsia is indistinguishable clinically or by EEG from other causes of generalized tonic-clonic seizures. Not all women with eclampsia require head imaging. However, if the seizure lasts >10 min, is recurrent, occurs postpartum or on seizure prophylaxis, or if there is evidence of localizing neurologic signs, head imaging is indicated. The differential diagnosis includes cerebrovascular accident (intracerebral hemorrhage, cerebral venous thrombosis), hypertensive encephalopathy, space-occupying lesions (brain tumor, abscess), metabolic disorders (hypoglycemia, uremia, inappropriate antidiuretic hormone secretion resulting in water intoxication), infectious etiology (meningitis, encephalitis), thrombotic thrombocytopenic purpura (TTP), and idiopathic epilepsy.

10. Eclampsia is an absolute contraindication to continued expectant management of severe pre-eclampsia. Immediate delivery is indicated regardless of gestational age. However, immediate delivery does not mean cesarean. Induction of labor and attempted vaginal delivery is a reasonable option, but prolonged induction of labor should be avoided. The decision about route of delivery should be individualized based on such factors as parity, gestational age, cervical examination (Bishop score), maternal desire for vaginal delivery, and fetal status and presentation. Regional anesthesia is preferred for women with eclampsia so long as close attention is paid to volume expansion and anesthetic technique, and there is no thrombocytopenia. Eclampsia always resolves following delivery although this may take a few days to weeks. Diuresis (>4 L/day) is the most accurate clinical indicator of resolving pre-eclampsia.

77 Shoulder Dystocia[1]

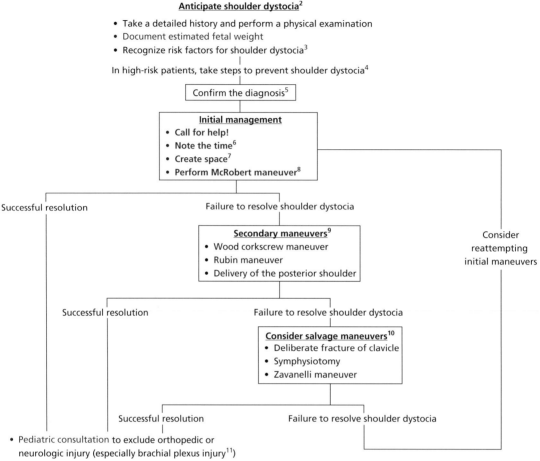

Anticipate shoulder dystocia[2]
- Take a detailed history and perform a physical examination
- Document estimated fetal weight
- Recognize risk factors for shoulder dystocia[3]

In high-risk patients, take steps to prevent shoulder dystocia[4]

Confirm the diagnosis[5]

Initial management
- **Call for help!**
- **Note the time[6]**
- **Create space[7]**
- **Perform McRobert maneuver[8]**

Successful resolution

Failure to resolve shoulder dystocia

Consider reattempting initial maneuvers

Secondary maneuvers[9]
- Wood corkscrew maneuver
- Rubin maneuver
- Delivery of the posterior shoulder

Successful resolution

Failure to resolve shoulder dystocia

Consider salvage maneuvers[10]
- Deliberate fracture of clavicle
- Symphysiotomy
- Zavanelli maneuver

Successful resolution

Failure to resolve shoulder dystocia

- Pediatric consultation to exclude orthopedic or neurologic injury (especially brachial plexus injury[11])
- Document events

1. Shoulder dystocia refers to impaction of the anterior shoulder of the fetus behind the pubic symphysis following delivery of the head. It is an obstetric emergency associated with neonatal birth trauma (neurologic injuries, fractures of the humerus, skull, clavicle) in up to 30% of cases. Shoulder dystocia complicates 0.2–2% of all vaginal deliveries. Immediate identification and prompt intervention may prevent neonatal birth trauma in some cases.

2. Although several risk factors for shoulder dystocia have been identified (see below), most cases occur in women with no risk factors. As such, it is not possible to accurately

Obstetric Clinical Algorithms: Management and Evidence. By © E.R. Norwitz, M. Belfort, G.R. Saade and H. Miller.
Published 2010 Blackwell Publishing.

predict all cases of shoulder dystocia. Obstetric care providers should be prepared to deal with shoulder dystocia at every vaginal delivery.

3. Risk factors for shoulder dystocia include a previous shoulder dystocia, fetal macrosomia, diabetes mellitus (including gestational diabetes), obesity, prolonged second stage of labor, precipitate labor, post-term pregnancy, and mid-cavity operative vaginal delivery.

4. Delivery management of women at risk of shoulder dystocia should be individualized. It may be prudent to deliver such patients in lithotomy position, to remove the bottom of the delivery bed to facilitate downward traction on the head, to pre-emptively empty the patient's bladder and (possibly) perform an episiotomy, and to have one or more experienced clinicians on hand. It may also be prudent to avoid operative vaginal deliveries in such patients.

5. Failure of the shoulders to deliver after delivery of the head should be noted immediately, especially if the head retracts into the birth canal ("turtle sign").

6. Delivery of the fetus within 5 minutes minimizes the risk of hypoxic ischemic injury.

7. If not already done, remove the bottom of the bed, empty the patient's bladder, and consider performing a generous episiotomy.

8. *McRobert maneuver* refers to hyperflexion of the patient's thighs onto her abdomen and suprapubic (not fundal) pressure. This maneuver does not increase the dimensions of the pelvis, but the cephalic rotation of the pelvis leads to a decrease in the angle of pelvic inclination, which frees the impacted anterior shoulder. This maneuver is successful in 60–80% of cases.

9. If McRobert maneuver is unsuccessful, a number of other maneuvers have been described. There is no proven advantage to any one of these. The decision of which to perform next should be left to the discretion and experience of the provider. These maneuvers include: (i) *Wood corkscrew maneuver* which is aimed at progressively rotating the posterior shoulder 180° in a corkscrew fashion to dislodge the anterior shoulder; (ii) *Rubin maneuver* in which pressure is applied laterally to the most accessible shoulder towards the anterior chest of the fetus with a view to

decreasing the bisacromial (shoulder-to-shoulder) diameter and freeing the impacted shoulder; and (iii) *delivery of the posterior shoulder* which consists of sweeping the posterior arm of the fetus across the chest, flexing the elbow manually, and delivering the posterior arm by traction on the wrist. This maneuver can result in fracture of the humerus, although humeral fractures usually heal without complication.

10. If these maneuvers are unsuccessful, "salvage" maneuvers can be attempted. These include: (i) *deliberate fracture of the anterior clavicle* which is performed manually by pushing the clavicle outwards against the ramus of the maternal pubis. The clavicle should not be fractured by pushing inwards towards the fetal chest since this can result in fetal pneumothorax or brachial plexus injury. In the absence of neurologic injury, the fracture will heal rapidly without incident; (ii) *symphysiotomy* consisting of surgical separation of the maternal pubic rami by transecting the cartilaginous symphysis pubis. It is very effective in expediting delivery, but is technically challenging and should not be attempted by inexperienced practitioners. It is associated with long-term nonunion and chronic severe pain to the mother. As such, it is rarely performed; (iii) *Zavanelli maneuver* which involves manual flexion and replacement of the fetal head back into the uterus followed by cesarean delivery. Reported success rates vary considerably.

11. Brachial plexus paralysis is the second most common neurologic birth injury (after facial nerve palsy) complicating 0.05–0.25% of all deliveries. It reportedly results from "excessive" lateral traction on the head and neck at delivery with resultant injury to the brachial plexus, usually to cervical nerve roots C5/C6 (Erb/Duchenne palsy). On examination, the arm hangs limply at the side of the body with the forearm extended and internally rotated, the classic "waiter's tip" deformity. The function of the fingers is usually retained. The lower brachial plexus (C8/T1) may also be involved resulting in paralysis of the hand, but isolated lower plexus injuries (Klumpke palsy) are rare. Ninety-five percent of brachial plexus injuries resolve completely within 2 years. Prognosis is especially good if recovery has started within 3 months. Elective cesarean delivery will prevent most (but not all) brachial plexus injuries. However, given the difficulty of predicting and preventing shoulder dystocia, cesarean delivery cannot be recommended for all women with identifiable risk factors.

78 Thyroid Storm

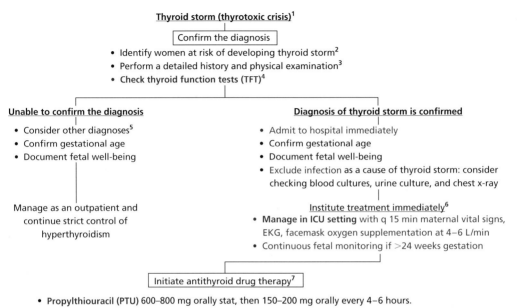

Thyroid storm (thyrotoxic crisis)[1]

Confirm the diagnosis

- Identify women at risk of developing thyroid storm[2]
- Perform a detailed history and physical examination[3]
- Check thyroid function tests (TFT)[4]

Unable to confirm the diagnosis

- Consider other diagnoses[5]
- Confirm gestational age
- Document fetal well-being

Manage as an outpatient and continue strict control of hyperthyroidism

Diagnosis of thyroid storm is confirmed

- Admit to hospital immediately
- Confirm gestational age
- Document fetal well-being
- Exclude infection as a cause of thyroid storm: consider checking blood cultures, urine culture, and chest x-ray

Institute treatment immediately[6]

- **Manage in ICU setting** with q 15 min maternal vital signs, EKG, facemask oxygen supplementation at 4–6 L/min
- Continuous fetal monitoring if >24 weeks gestation

Initiate antithyroid drug therapy[7]

- **Propylthiouracil (PTU)** 600–800 mg orally stat, then 150–200 mg orally every 4–6 hours. If oral administration is not possible, use methimazole rectal suppositories
- Starting 1–2 hours after PTU, administer **saturated solution of potassium iodide (SSKI)** 2–5 drops orally every 8 hours. Alternative sources of iodine may include sodium iodide (0.5–1.0 g iv every 8 hours) or Lugol solution (8 drops every 6 hours) or lithium carbonate (300 mg orally every 6 hours)
- **Dexamethasone** 2 mg iv or im every 6 hours for four doses
- **Propranolol** 20–80 mg orally every 4–6 hours or 1–2 mg iv every 5 minutes for a total of 6 mg, then 1–10 mg iv every 4 hours. If the patient has a history of severe bronchospasm, consider reserpine (1–5 mg im every 4–6 hours) or guanethidine (1 mg/kg orally every 12 hours) or diltiazem (60 mg orally every 6–8 hours)
- Phenobarbital 30–60 mg orally every 6–8 hours as needed for extreme restlessness

Once the patient is stable, continue close observation[8]

Obstetric Clinical Algorithms: Management and Evidence. By © E.R. Norwitz, M. Belfort, G.R. Saade and H. Miller.
Published 2010 Blackwell Publishing.

1. Thyroid storm (thyrotoxic crisis) is a medical emergency characterized by a severe acute exacerbation of the signs and symptoms of hyperthyroidism. It is a rare complication, occurring in approximately 1% of pregnant patients with hyperthyroidism, but is associated with significant maternal and perinatal mortality and morbidity.

2. The vast majority of women presenting with thyroid storm have a history of hyperthyroidism. Hyperthyroidism refers to the clinical state resulting from an excess production of and exposure to thyroid hormone. The most common cause is Graves disease, which accounts for 95% of all cases of hyperthyroidism in pregnancy and is caused by circulating thyroid-stimulating autoantibodies. Ophthalmopathy (lid lag, lid retraction) and dermopathy (pretibial edema) are clinical signs that are specific to Graves disease. Other causes include inflammation (thyroiditis), toxic multinodular goiter, solitary toxic thyroid nodule, hyperemesis gravidarum/gestational trophoblastic neoplasia, exogenous thyroid hormone, and a TSH-secreting pituitary adenoma. In order to minimize complications (including thyroid storm), hyperthyroidism is best diagnosed and treated prior to pregnancy. An inciting event (such as infection, hypoglycemia, diabetic ketoacidosis, venous thromboembolism, surgery, and/or labor and delivery) can be identified in many instances of thyroid storm.

3. Thyroid storm is diagnosed by a combination of symptoms and signs in patients with thyrotoxicosis, including fever, tachycardia out of proportion to the fever >140–160 bpm, altered mental status (such as restlessness, nervousness, confusion or seizures), diarrhea, vomiting, and cardiac arrhythmia. However, the diagnosis can be difficult to make clinically.

4. If thyroid storm is suspected, serum TFT should be sent immediately. Biochemical findings supportive of the diagnosis include suppressed levels of thyroid-binding globulin (<0.05 mU/mL) and increased free levothyroxine (T_4) and L-triiodithyronine (T_3) in the maternal circulation. Although most women with Graves disease will have circulating anti-TSH receptor, antimicrosomal, and/or antithyroid peroxidase autoantibodies, measurement of such antibodies is neither required nor recommended to establish the diagnosis. Moreover, antibody levels do not correlate with either maternal or perinatal outcome.

5. The differential diagnosis of thyroid storm includes anxiety disorders, drug intoxication and/or withdrawal, and pheochromocytoma.

6. Thyroid storm is associated with significant maternal and perinatal mortality and morbidity, including shock, stupor, coma, and death. If the clinical index of suspicion for thyroid storm is high, treatment should be initiated immediately and should not be withheld pending the results of biochemical tests.

7. The goals of treatment of thyroid storm are: (i) to reduce the synthesis and release of hormone from the thyroid gland using thioamides (such as PTU) or methimazole, supplemental iodide, and glucocorticoids; (ii) to block the peripheral actions of thyroid hormones using glucocorticoids, PTU, and high-dose β-blockers; (iii) to treat complications and support physiologic functions (manage in an ICU setting, acetaminophen, cooling blankets, supplemental oxygen, fluid and caloric replacement); and (iv) to identify and treat precipitating events (such as hypoglycemia, thromboembolic events, and diabetic ketoacidosis). As with other acute maternal illnesses, fetal well-being should be appropriately evaluated and consideration given to delivery, if appropriate. Fetal tachycardia (>160 bpm) is a sensitive index of fetal hyperthyroidism. Only 1–5% of neonates born to women with poorly controlled thyrotoxicosis will develop transient hyperthyroidism or neonatal Graves disease caused by the transplacental passage of maternal antithyroid antibodies.

8. Once stable, it is important to: (i) follow serum electrolytes (especially K^+) and arterial blood gas q 2–4 hourly, as indicated; (ii) catheterize patient if unconscious or not passing urine; (iii) aspirate and decompress stomach if unconscious; and (iv) continue fetal surveillance and consideration for delivery, if indicated. For women who fail to respond to initial medical therapy, options are limited. Radioactive iodine (^{131}I) administration to ablate the thyroid gland is absolutely contraindicated in pregnancy. Surgery is best avoided, but may be required.

Index